Diabetes
Beating the Odds

Diabetes
Beating the Odds

The Doctor's Guide
to Reducing Your Risk

Elliot J. Rayfield, M.D.
Cheryl Solimini

Illustrations by Mona Mark

Addison-Wesley Publishing Company
Reading, Massachusetts • Menlo Park, California
New York • Don Mills, Ontario • Wokingham, England
Amsterdam • Bonn • Madrid • San Juan • Paris • Seoul
Milan • Mexico City • Taipei

Many of the designations used by manufacturers and sellers to distinguish their products are claimed as trademarks. Where those designations appear in this book and Addison-Wesley was aware of a trademark claim, the designations have been printed in initial capital letters (i.e., NutraSweet).

Library of Congress Cataloging-in-Publication Data

Rayfield, Elliot J.
  Diabetes—beating the odds : the doctor's guide to reducing your risk / Elliot J. Rayfield, Cheryl Solimini ; illustrations by Mona Mark.
    p.   cm.
  Includes index.
  ISBN 0-201-57784-4
  1. Diabetes—Popular works. 2. Diabetes—Prevention. 3. Diabetes—Risk factors. I. Solimini, Cheryl. II. Title.
RC660.4.R38   1992
616.4'62—dc20   92-14725
                                                             CIP

Cover design by John Martucci
Text design by Joyce C. Weston
Set in 10-point Clarendon by NK Graphics, Keene, NH

1 2 3 4 5 6 7 8 9-MU-95949392
First printing, October 1992

Contents

List of Illustrations

Acknowledgments

We would like to thank Cathy Piuggi, R.D., C.D.E. and Richard W. Weil, M.Ed., C.D.E. for their valuable contributions to Chapters Five and Six, respectively. We also appreciate the help and cooperation of the American Diabetes Association.

Diabetes
Beating the Odds

1

The Genetic Connection: How Diabetes Runs in the Family

WHEN any family gathers together, it's easy to see where heredity has left its mark: a brother and sister with the same curly red hair, a set of dimples that seems to have been passed down from one generation to the next, a child's wide smile reflected in her grandmother's. To hear "He looks just like his Dad" is a source of pride to most fathers, and surely one of the great joys of parenthood is recognizing a part of yourself or a loved one in your children.

However, unlike curly hair or green eyes, other traits that we inherit are not so obvious—or as desirable. Many diseases can also be traced along family lines, and diabetes mellitus (usually just called diabetes) is one of them.

If you've picked up this book, you probably have diabetes or have a close relative who has diabetes or had it at some point. Perhaps the knowledge that a parent died of diabetes or its many complications is already a concern in your life. Perhaps you worry that the same fate awaits you or your children, and you feel that developing the disease is an ever-present threat to your family's future.

These thoughts can be frightening, but they needn't be. Yes, diabetes is a serious, often life-threatening disorder that can affect generations of the same family. And it's true that our genes are responsible for much of what we are and what we will become. The appropriate combination of genes calling for curly hair and green eyes will create curly hair and green eyes. But not all genes express themselves this directly. Just because an illness runs in the family does not mean that illness is inevitable—a fate to be awaited passively. What you inherit is a *predisposition* to some diseases. In fact, some other factor may be the trigger that makes the *possibility* of illness a *reality*. Your best defense is to learn as much as you can about the disease and what causes it. That includes probing into your relatives' backgrounds and taking a closer look at what you might be doing to put yourself at risk.

This is the case with diabetes. One out of every five children born today will be vulnerable to this disease. Because evidence indicates that diabetes is inherited, scientists know that a specific gene or a combination of genes are responsible—but they have yet to find the gene or genes that pass on this tendency and who within each generation will get it. However, tremendous strides have been made in the past 20 years in trying to detect who is at risk. Medical researchers do know that diabetes is one of many genetic disorders that may be "switched on" by certain conditions in a person's life-style or environment.

It's these factors that you *can* control. By making changes in specific aspects of your life, you can ward off diabetes altogether, delay its onset, or at the very least lessen the severity of the disease and its possible complications.

Before you undertake the program of changes that will be explained in later chapters, you should be aware that there are several forms of diabetes, each with different causes and consequences. Once you determine which type is common to your family, you can better know how to take action. But first you should have a general understanding of the disorder and its development, so you will see how taking action will help you and your family beat the odds against diabetes.

WHAT IS DIABETES?

The disease's major symptom—passing large amounts of urine—has been a part of recorded medical history since about 1500 B.C. The Greeks had a name for it: *diabetes*, meaning "siphon" or "flowing through." Centuries later, when it was discovered that the urine had a sweet taste, the Latin *mellitus* ("honey-like") was added.

Only in the late 1700s did scientists determine that the sweetness is caused by excess glucose—also called blood sugar—overflowing into the urine. It took another 200 years before the problem was traced to the pancreas, a six-inch-long, comma-shaped gland that sits behind and beneath the stomach (see Figure 1): In 1889 Joseph von Mering and Oskar Minkowski removed the mysterious gland from dogs, who quickly developed diabetes-like symptoms.

We now know that the pancreas is responsible for several aspects of food metabolism. It produces enzymes that aid in the digestion of starches and protein. It also contains the *islets of Langerhans,* named after the German scientist who discovered them in 1869 (see Figure 2). Located primarily in the pancreas's "tail," these clusters of cells manufacture protein-like *hormones*—the special chemicals that are released into the bloodstream to regulate the behavior of other cells or organs. Within the islets are *alpha cells*, which manufacture glucagon that raises the amount of glucose in the blood; *beta cells*, the producers of insulin, which lowers glucose levels; *delta cells*, which make somatostatin, a hormone that has several functions, including inhibiting insulin and releasing glucagon from the islets and growth hormone from the pituitary gland; and *pancreatic polypeptide cells*, which secrete pancreatic polypeptide and about which little is known.

Finally insulin—or rather, the lack of it—was identified

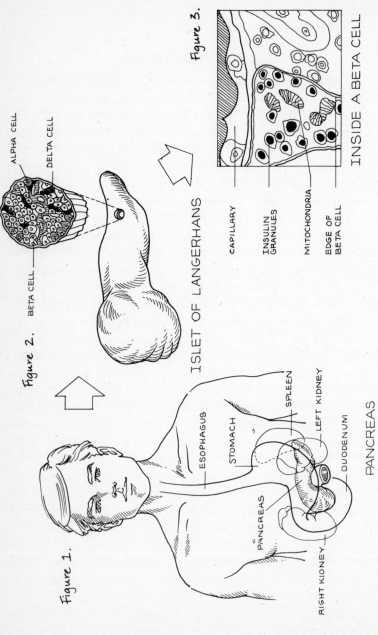

Figure 1.

Figure 2.

Figure 3.

PANCREAS

ESOPHAGUS

STOMACH

SPLEEN

LEFT KIDNEY

DUODENUM

PANCREAS

RIGHT KIDNEY

ISLET OF LANGERHANS

ALPHA CELL

DELTA CELL

BETA CELL

INSIDE A BETA CELL

CAPILLARY

INSULIN GRANULES

MITOCHONDRIA

EDGE OF BETA CELL

as the main culprit in diabetes mellitus. In 1922 insulin extracted from animals was injected into a young boy with diabetes and brought about his dramatic recovery. With that, it was assumed the search for a "cure" for diabetes was over. Until then, those who had developed diabetes were doomed to an early death.

While the treatment did prolong countless lives, several decades passed before scientists realized that an injection of insulin did not offer a permanent solution. It was not effective in every case. For those it helped, blood-sugar levels still had to be carefully monitored and insulin given at the right times. And insulin alone did not prevent the complications that eventually affected patients: damage to vision, kidneys, nerves, and blood vessels. Only within the last 20 years or so have doctors become aware that those with diabetes need to regulate more than their blood glucose: diet, exercise, and a reduction in stress would be necessary for the patient with diabetes to live as normally as possible.

At the root of diabetes mellitus is the beta cells' inability to produce any or enough insulin (see Figure 3), or else whatever insulin is available cannot be used by the body. To understand how insulin is implicated in diabetes, you need to look at the entire metabolic process—how our systems receive and use food for energy.

Everything we eat can be divided into three fuel sources: carbohydrates, proteins, and fats. Once in the digestive system, they are broken down by stomach enzymes into glucose, amino acids, and fatty acids, respectively.

The body's *first choice* for energy is glucose. Readily available in the bloodstream, glucose comes from carbohydrates—complex ones like starches (breads, potatoes, whole grains, fruits, and vegetables) and simple ones like sucrose (table sugar) and fructose (honey). The *second-best fuel*—protein—comes from meat, seafood, dairy products, legumes (peas, beans), and nuts; it's used to build muscle and bone. In order to be used for energy, protein must first be converted to amino acids, which can then be changed into glucose in the liver and stored there or in the muscles. (Stored glucose is called *glycogen.*) Fats—found in butter, lard, vegetable oils, meats, and dairy foods—are necessary for healthy skin and the absorption of some vitamins, and are the last and least efficient energy source.

Once glucose is in the bloodstream, it tries to enter the individual cells to nourish them. But it can't get in without a key—and that key is insulin (see Figure 4). On each cell's surface sit many insulin receptors—they're the "keyholes" that insulin molecules fit into to open the way for glucose. Insulin sends the signal for nearby glucose transporters to open up and take in glucose, so it penetrates the outer membrane of each cell. (Insulin's signal also triggers other activities within cells that are necessary for their growth.)

Trouble starts when the pancreas is not producing enough insulin or if for some reason the cells are resisting whatever insulin there may be. Unable to get inside cells, the glucose remains in the bloodstream and the blood's sugar level builds up—a condition called *hyperglycemia.*

There is always some sugar in the blood. Usually, extra glucose is stored in the liver as glycogen, or it is kept in reserve in the muscles for times when sudden physical exertion is required. When these warehouses are filled, the body turns to storage space that has no limits: the fat cells. (When the body must tap into these reserves, glucagon is released from the pancreatic alpha cells and epinephrine is released from the inner compartment of the adrenal glands to break the glycogen back down into glucose.) But in every case, insulin is needed to convert glucose into a storable form.

Without insulin, the liver, muscle, and fat cells are deprived of their energy source. Weak and fatigued, the body thinks it is starving and signals extreme hunger (*polyphagia*). When glucose can't be used for fuel, the body seeks

THE ACTION OF INSULIN AND GLUCOSE IN A CELL

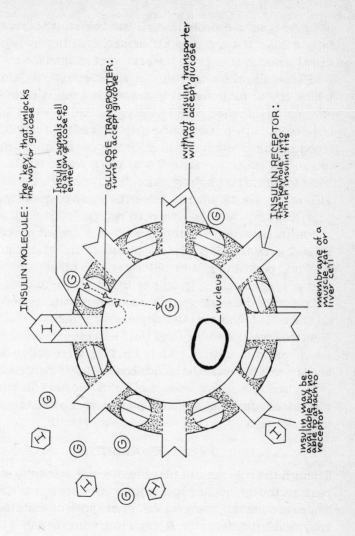

INSULIN MOLECULE: the "key" that unlocks the way for glucose

Insulin signals cell to allow glucose to enter

GLUCOSE TRANSPORTER: turns to accept glucose

without insulin, transporter will not accept glucose

INSULIN RECEPTOR: the "lock" into which insulin fits

membrane of a muscle, fat or liver cell

insulin may be available but not attach to receptor

nucleus

out glycogen and protein. As a last resort, it burns stored fatty acids—but not very efficiently, creating by-products called ketones that raise the acid level in the blood.

Meanwhile, the sugar-loaded blood enters the kidneys, which try to filter useful glucose and keep it from being eliminated into the urine. However, the kidneys can retrieve only so much glucose; once they've reached their limit (a blood sugar of over 180 mg/dl), the sugar spills into the urine. Too much sugar in the urine (*glycosuria*) alerts the body to dilute it, sending more fluids through the kidney. This is why people with diabetes urinate so frequently (*polyuria*) and why they are always thirsty (*polydipsia*): the body is continually dehydrating. Also lost in the elimination of these fluids are electrolytes—dissolved minerals (such as sodium, potassium, and chloride) and other compounds that are essential for good health. In severe diabetes, urination may cease altogether as the circulating blood and all the cells become totally depleted of fluids.

As this cycle of energy and fluid loss progresses, the body must continue to turn to fats for fuel. Gradually the acid level from ketones in the blood becomes too high, developing into a toxic condition known as *ketoacidosis*. This can lead to nausea, vomiting, stomach pain, deep labored breathing, or, if not treated, a diabetic coma—and death.

TYPES OF DIABETES

Though the role insulin plays in diabetes is easy to see, the reasons the metabolic process goes awry are not so obvious. There are actually several different types of diabetes, and they develop differently. It's extremely important to look at these distinct forms in order to determine your own inherited risk and what can be done to prevent it.

The major forms are Type I and Type II. Nearly all the diagnosed cases of diabetes fall into one of these two groups.

Type I

Type I used to be known as juvenile diabetes because it typically strikes children and adolescents. We now know it is possible for Type I to develop after age 20, so today it is more accurately called insulin-dependent diabetes mellitus (IDDM). Though Type I is less common—it accounts for only about 5 to 10 percent of 14 million diabetes cases in the United States and is the most severe form. It usually develops more suddenly than Type II diabetes—within a few days or weeks. Sometimes a person first learns of the disease after having been rushed to the hospital with ketoacidosis. However, in the last several years, researchers have learned that the onset of Type I diabetes in many cases may develop months or years before symptoms are noticeable.

Because their own pancreases manufacture no, or very little, insulin, IDDM patients must depend on daily injections of the hormone to stay alive. (Insulin cannot be taken orally.) They must be vigilant in keeping track of blood-sugar levels and in administering appropriate doses of insulin; the goal is to try to duplicate normal, stable blood-sugar levels as closely as possible. Careful eating, regular exercise, and stress reduction are also necessary to control the disorder.

Type I diabetes is generally considered to be a malfunction of the body's immune system. In IDDM, the lack of insulin stems from destruction of the beta cells. Scientific evidence points to another factor—in some cases, a virus—that may have invaded the cells, forcing the body to produce antibodies to fight it. (These antibodies have been found in the bloodstreams of Type I patients.) The antibodies, sent in to destroy the infection, instead wind up destroying the beta cells themselves.

Though Type I does tend to run in families, the pattern of inheritance is far from clear—or strong. Studies of identical twins indicate that if one has IDDM before age 20, the other has close to a 50 percent chance of developing it too. Other siblings of an IDDM patient have a greater risk for diabetes than the general population. If they share certain pieces of genetic material (HLA antigens—discussed below), their risk is 20 percent; if not, their chance of developing IDDM is much smaller: about 5 to 10 percent. The disorder also seems to follow paternal lines: children whose fathers have Type I diabetes appear to be five times more likely to develop it than children whose mothers have the disease. But 85 percent of all cases of IDDM occur without an immediate-family history of the disease. It may be that the illness skips generations or is the result of other factors that can be traced to the person's environment—for instance, toxins, chemicals, viruses, nutritional factors, and stress.

The theory is that someone does not directly inherit Type I diabetes but rather the susceptibility to it. Actually, what may be passed down is the vulnerability to the viral infection that attacks the beta cells. Evidence for this theory has been gathered by examining IDDM patients for the presence of particular groups of infection-fighters: *human leukocyte antigens* (HLA). Scientists believe that these are one set of

Relative Risk for Type I Diabetes

If you have . . .	Your risk is:
A diabetic twin	1 in 3
Another sibling who is diabetic	1 in 14
One parent who is diabetic	1 in 25
Your mother is the diabetic parent	1 in 40–50
Your father is the diabetic parent	1 in 20
No diabetic relative	1 in 500

SOURCE: J.I. Rotter; E.M. Landaw; N. Maclaren, et al., *Diabetes,* 1983; 32:75A.

genetic markers that show if someone is at risk for Type I diabetes. Here's how the HLA groups are involved:

Every human cell has 23 pairs of chromosomes, and each pair carries the genes that determine our physical traits. (Each pair of chromosomes has the same genes as all the other pairs.) Produced by genes located on Chromosome 6, the HLA antigens are proteins that sit on the cell surfaces to fight illness. Scientists have divided these antigens into five groups—A, B, C, D, and DR (meaning D-related)—and the genes determine what combination of these groups, out of the many possible variations, each person will get.

Though several HLA groups have been implicated in Type I diabetes, researchers have found that 90 percent of all children with IDDM have DR3 or DR4. Any person with HLA-DR4 or HLA-DR3 is considered to be five to eight times more likely to develop IDDM; if both groups are present, there's a 20-to-40-times higher risk. And some antigen groups may actually protect against diabetes: people with HLA-DR2 have an extremely low risk.

In family studies, a sibling who has all the same HLA types as a diabetic brother or sister has the highest risk— 12 to 24 percent—of developing IDDM. If they share only one HLA type, the risk drops to 4 to 7 percent, and to 1 to 2 percent if no HLA types are similar.

But the HLA-DR system may not be the only—or the best—genetic marker. Recently researchers have been able to test for another HLA system, the DQ group, that has a high association with IDDM. In fact, they think the DQ has more promise than the DR in predicting who is susceptible to Type I diabetes (Figure 5). They concluded that the presence of an antigen they call DQw1.2 had a protective effect and that having DQw8 increased the risk. Much more work needs to be done to more clearly understand all the factors involved in the DQ group.

Still, pinpointing who will eventually develop IDDM by

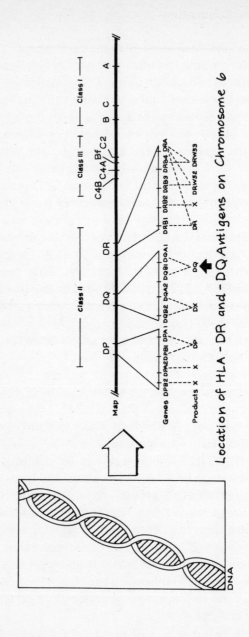

Location of HLA-DR and-DQ Antigens on Chromosome 6

looking for specific HLA groups is not practical at this time. About 50 percent of the nonaffected population has one or a combination of the HLA-DR antigens, and 98 percent will never develop diabetes. What the finding of antigens common to Type I may lead to is the discovery of yet another antigen or a combination of antigens that scientists can count on to predict the disease. Knowing which gene is responsible may make it possible to correct the defective gene before diabetes can develop.

Though they have yet to find a way to detect diabetes before the fact, researchers have uncovered a method that points to the disease's development before the most obvious signs appear. They can check to see if a person's blood contains the beta-cell-attacking antibodies, which are present months, sometimes years, before diabetes strikes. (Approximately 80 percent of Type I patients were found to have these antibodies at the time they were diagnosed.) Studies are now under way to determine if, by treating people at this stage in the disease, IDDM can be prevented from ever developing further.

Type II

Type II, or non-insulin-dependent diabetes mellitus (NIDDM), makes up the majority—90 to 95 percent—of diabetes cases known around the world. In the United States, it is estimated that about 13 million people have Type II. This is only an estimate, because medical experts believe that for every NIDDM case diagnosed, there is at least one other case that goes undiagnosed. Unlike Type I, whose symptoms usually are much more dramatic and require immediate medical attention, Type II progresses more slowly; those with NIDDM might not seek treatment until the complications of the disease—such as vision problems or numbness in the feet—show themselves. NIDDM usually occurs after age 40, which is why until recently it was called adult-onset diabetes. However, it can also develop before age 25, when it is classified as MODY (maturity-onset diabetes of the young).

Unlike those with Type I, people who have Type II diabetes *are* producing their own insulin—sometimes even more than enough. But for some reason their bodies are resistant to it. This may be because there are too few receptors on the outside of cells to accept the insulin, or the receptors may be defective and the insulin cannot bind as efficiently. Sometimes the glucose may enter but the cells may fail to use it. Or too little insulin may be available because of a reduction in beta cells. In less than 0.5 percent of NIDDM cases, "mutant insulin"—an abnormal, less potent form of the hormone—was found to be the culprit. Whatever the cause, the glucose cannot nourish the cell sufficiently.

However, the consequences are different from those of Type I. People with Type II diabetes are usually not prone to ketoacidosis, unless subjected to a great deal of stress. NIDDM patients usually do not need to inject more insulin; some may need to take other drugs orally that help the cells overcome insulin resistance. But often the simplest and safest way to control Type II is to lose weight. No one is quite sure why, but excess fat seems to hamper the body's sensitivity to insulin. About 60 to 80 percent of people diagnosed with Type II in Western countries are obese—20 percent or more above their ideal weight.

NIDDM has a strong family connection (see chart below). In studies of identical twins, it was found that if after age 40 one twin has Type II diabetes, the other has a nearly 100 percent chance of developing it. (Before age 40, it's 50 percent.) If another brother or sister has NIDDM, the risk is about 30 percent. If one parent has Type II, an offspring has a 35 percent chance of having it later in life; the risk doubles when both parents have diabetes.

MODY draws an even stronger line to heredity. In one study, 85 percent of these young patients had at least one parent with diabetes, 53 percent of their siblings were

MODYs, and 46 percent had a diabetic grandparent—three generations of diabetes!

Despite an obvious inheritance pattern, researchers are still working on reliable genetic markers for Type II. Dr. Alan Permutt and associates have recently identified a glucokinase gene as a genetic marker for NIDDM in American blacks. NIDDM is not associated with specific HLA antigens or with the presence of antibodies in the blood. Scientists suspect that molecules called *islet amyloid polypeptides,* found in the islets of Langerhans and common to those with NIDDM, may be interfering with insulin's action. But whether amyloid peptides are just a part of the progress of diabetes or are its cause needs further study. So, for now, tracing a family history and screening for other risk factors (which you'll learn more about in Chapter 2) is the closest science can come to predicting who will get Type II.

Occasionally doctors may have difficulty in classifying a case of diabetes as either Type I or Type II. For instance, most Type I patients are thin, but so are some Type IIs. Someone with the characteristics of NIDDM may actually need insulin therapy to control blood sugar, though he or she is not dependent on it to live. The problem of an inaccurate diagnosis may rest on finding a way to measure

Percentage of Diabetic Offspring, by Diabetic Status of the Parent, United States, 1976-1980

Age of Index Offspring (Years)	Both Parents Diabetic	Only Mother Diabetic	Only Father Diabetic	Neither Diabetic
20–34	5.8	2.1	2.0	0.7
35–44	7.3	3.6	3.2	1.1
45–54	10.5	5.8	8.0	2.9
55–64	25.5	9.6	13.2	3.7
65–74	21.5	11.3	11.7	4.6

SOURCE: Maureen I. Harris, National Diabetes Data Group, from data of the 1976–80 National Health and Nutrition Survey, National Center for Health Statistics.

insulin secretion, which scientists are not able to do on a patient who is taking insulin injections. However, they can measure the levels of C-peptides. (Beta cells actually first produce a substance called *proinsulin,* which then divides into two smaller units—creating insulin and C-peptides. Unlike insulin, these peptides remain only in the bloodstream, and seem to serve no biological purpose.) Testing for C-peptides has helped greatly in distinguishing between the two types, and in the future may be used to predict if a Type II patient will require insulin eventually.

Gestational Diabetes

Gestational diabetes describes a diabetic condition, or glucose intolerance, that develops or is first detected during pregnancy. (This category does not include anyone who was known to have diabetes *before* becoming pregnant.) Women who have a family history of any type of diabetes face a greater risk of gestational diabetes. It affects about 2 percent of all pregnant women, usually in the second or third trimester. Normally at that point in the pregnancy, the placenta begins releasing hormones that interfere with insulin. Diabetes results when the woman cannot produce enough insulin to keep blood-sugar levels steady.

Usually gestational diabetes can be controlled through a strict diet. But if the illness is not carefully managed, the fetus takes up the extra glucose and grows abnormally large—a danger to the child and the mother. After delivery, the baby may suffer low blood sugar (*hypoglycemia*) because it has become accustomed to receiving both its own and its mother's glucose.

Since diabetes can be harmful to the fetus, every woman should be screened between the 24th and 28th weeks of pregnancy. Most women with gestational diabetes that has been adequately treated will return to normal following delivery. However, 60 percent will develop diabetes, most often Type II, within 15 years after giving birth. Some animal studies have shown that a female with glucose intolerance during pregnancy can pass the tendency on to her offspring, who will develop diabetes some time later in their lives.

Secondary Diabetes

Secondary diabetes can occur when other conditions affect either the body's ability to handle glucose or its production of insulin. For instance, secondary diabetes may be triggered by malnutrition, some types of drugs or chemicals, or a defect of the insulin receptors. It can develop in people who have had their pancreases removed, or who suffer from a disease of the pancreas (such as cystic fibrosis) or of another endocrine gland (Cushing's syndrome). Genetic syndromes, such as muscular dystrophy and Huntington's chorea, are also associated with this form of diabetes. But the diabetes itself has no direct connection to family inheritance; therefore it is not a type that can be adequately predicted, nor can it be prevented without eliminating the primary cause of illness.

Impaired Glucose Tolerance

Impaired glucose tolerance (IGT)—formerly called borderline or chemical diabetes—is not a true form of diabetes, but it may be an early stage of Type I or, more often, Type II. It is diagnosed when blood-sugar levels are higher than normal, but not high enough to be classified as diabetes mellitus. The National Diabetes Data Group estimates that between 7 and 18 million Americans between ages 20 and 74 have IGT. While it doesn't carry the same complications as diabetes, IGT does seem to increase the risk for heart disease. Studies show that within 10 years of being diagnosed with IGT, anywhere from 10 to 50 percent of patients develop Type II.

*   *   *

When investigating diabetes, researchers also use two other terms: *previous abnormality of glucose tolerance* (prev AGT) and *potential abnormality of glucose tolerance* (pot AGT). *Prev AGT* describes anyone who has tested positive for diabetes mellitus or impaired glucose tolerance in the past but whose blood-sugar levels are currently within the normal range. This category also includes women who have had gestational diabetes, formerly obese NIDDM patients whose glucose levels returned to normal once they had lost weight, Type I patients with diabetes temporarily in remission (a rare occurrence), and those whose sugar levels rose after a one-time trauma—such as surgery or third-degree burns. *Pot AGT* subjects have never had elevated levels of blood glucose but they are under observation because they have a family history of diabetes, have HLA-DR3 or -DR4 antigens or islet-cell antibodies, or are obese, or gave birth to unusually large babies. Statistically, people classified as prev AGT or pot AGT are more likely to develop diabetes in the future. However, these terms are used only by scientists to identify certain at-risk individuals—and are not considered to be a diagnosis of disease.

IS GENETIC COUNSELING WORTHWHILE?

Once you have recognized the type of diabetes that runs in your family, you might be concerned about how this heredity will affect you and future generations. Should the risk of passing on a "diabetes gene" influence whom you marry or whether you should have children?

Unlike carrying the gene for a more devastating disease like sickle-cell anemia, cystic fibrosis, or Tay-Sachs, the inheritance factor in diabetes would not doom a child to a diminished quality of life—mental retardation, a crippling birth defect, or debilitating illness. Certainly diabetes is a serious disorder, but if managed well, it should not interfere with living normally, though with some restrictions. If you already have diabetes and become pregnant, your condition does pose some risks to you and your fetus. But that is another issue: the problems evolve from the environment of the womb and the stress that diabetes places on the body; it is not related to genetics.

The truth is that most fear passing on or inheriting Type I diabetes because of its more severe consequences, yet the evidence reasssures us that the overall risk to first-degree relatives of an IDDM patient is low. And treatment for Type I has come a long way from the days before insulin was available, when half of the children diagnosed with the disease died within one year of onset; today that risk is about one percent. For Type II, most people will not know if they have the disorder until their childbearing years are over, so the information for calculating the risk to offspring would probably be incomplete at the time of marriage or family planning.

The latest research is bringing us closer to a genetic marker that may indicate definitely who will develop diabetes, which will perhaps bring us closer to a cure. But at this time, a genetic counselor cannot offer the kind of specific guidance that is possible for other conditions. Still, a counselor could provide you with an approximate risk based on currently available information.

You might talk over any concerns with your family physician. She or he can ask you specific questions about family history and other factors, such as those that will be discussed in the next chapter, that might put you and your offspring at risk. If you already have children, you will want to discuss their risk based on what you know of the diabetes background in both your and your spouse's families; talking to older relatives can turn up clues to help trace the disease pattern. If you have not started a family of your own but plan to do so, you should explore the risks now, to see what you can do to minimize the chances of encouraging a genetic susceptibility to diabetes. Your doc-

tor may suggest that you seek the advice of a genetic counselor depending on how clear-cut your family history and
that of your spouse are.

Learn as much as you can about diabetes and encourage
your children to do so. This book is meant to start you in
the right direction. The following chapters include information on other risk factors involved in the development of
diabetes, the early warning signs of the disease, and the
tests that can mean early detection—and a chance of slowing or stopping diabetes' progress. But most important are
the suggestions for life-style changes that can head off diabetes before it ever takes hold.

All the evidence indicates that the most effective ways to
control diabetes are to pay attention to diet, schedule regular moderate exercise, and avoid situations that create
stress. These same strategies can help you beat the odds
against diabetes. Here you'll find the guidance you'll need
for proper nutrition and healthful weight loss, how to plan
a fitness routine that you can stick with, and techniques
for lessening stress's impact. With these tools, you may be
able to eliminate completely the threat of diabetes to you
and your family.

CHAPTER
2

Are You Adding to Your Risk?: Factors You Can Control

AS you learned from the preceding chapter, heredity alone doesn't determine who will get diabetes. In fact, many other elements—one or a combination—may influence whether an individual with an inherited predisposition to the disease will actually develop it. Your complete pattern of genes (genotype) is set from birth, but certain traits make their appearance only because the environment acts in certain ways on these genes.

By this standard, your chances of preventing Type II diabetes—or certainly of delaying its onset and lessening its impact—are excellent. For Type I, the mechanisms that set it off are more complex and less able to be controlled, but the latest research offers more hope that it, too, can be headed off before it develops.

Some of the characteristics and circumstances, other than heredity, that are common to diabetes are discussed here. (As before, Type I and Type II are treated separately, because they are different diseases.) Make note of which risk factors apply to you or other family members. You will see that some elements—obesity in Type II, for instance, or exposure to viruses for Type I—can be eliminated or avoided, lowering the odds of developing diabetes. Others, such as eth-

nic origins, obviously cannot be altered. But knowing that
these unalterable factors are in your background makes it
even more vital for you to do something about what you
can change.

TYPE I RISK FACTORS

Age: If you're already over 40 years old, there's little chance
that you will be stricken with Type I diabetes. However, if
you have young children and there's a family history of
IDDM, you should remain alert to signs of the disease in
them. As mentioned earlier, most cases of IDDM occur in
children and adolescents; after 20 years of age, any risk for
Type I is cut in half. In girls, the peak period for the onset
of the disease is around 12 to 13 years old; for boys, one to
two years later. Exactly when Type I strikes may be related
to which HLA type a child has. With IDDM that surfaces in
adults, the pattern is not known, because there is so little
accurate information about it.

The mother's age at time of her child's birth may also play
a part: children with IDDM were twice as likely to have been
born to women over age 35. Why is not clear, but it may be
linked to the mother's own glucose tolerance, which naturally declines with aging; this may somehow affect the environment of the womb.

Gender: Though statistics vary, there seems to be little difference between males and females in risk of Type I diabetes.

Race: Only a few studies have compared the risk for different ethnic origins. In the United States, two Pennsylvania
studies indicated that whites are one and a half times more
likely than blacks to have IDDM. Hispanic children—at
least this was true in Colorado and in San Diego—are less
at risk than white youngsters. Among American Indians,

the few cases of IDDM primarily strike those of mixed heritage. Canadian research showed that children from British and Jewish backgrounds were at 50 percent greater risk than those of French or Italian ancestry. In New Zealand, children of European origin were three times more likely to have IDDM than youngsters of Polynesian descent. This seems to indicate an inherited risk among some ethnic groups.

Socioeconomic Status: The relation between family income and diabetes hasn't been clearly established—and is mainly conflicting. In England and Montreal, IDDM occurred twice as often in children from higher social classes. But in Copenhagen higher rates were reported for poorer youngsters. A Pennsylvania study showed no difference between socioeconomic groups.

Season: Those susceptible to IDDM may be more vulnerable at certain times of year. In the Northern and Western hemispheres, new cases seem to appear most often in the fall and winter months—perhaps because that is when common viral infections are more active. (Read more about viruses, below.)

Geography: Cooler climates seem to breed more IDDM patients. Each year in Finland 29.5 children per 100,000 are diagnosed with IDDM, the highest rate in Europe. Norway, Sweden, and Scotland also have high rates of incidence. (Japan has the lowest: 1.7 per 100,000.) However, Sardinia also has an extremely high incidence of diabetes which cannot be explained on the basis of geography. In the United States, Rochester, Minnesota, has a rate of 20.8, while warmer San Diego comes in at 9.4. Perhaps the cold lowers immunity to a virus that triggers IDDM—that might also explain the seasonal incidence. However, no real conclusions can be drawn because these studies have not eliminated other factors, such as ethnic origins or diet, that might also be common to these regions.

Viruses: As mentioned in Chapter 1, some cases of IDDM have been linked to exposure to a virus that might switch on the autoimmune response that destroys insulin-producing beta cells. In fact, scientists have identified several infections that are associated with the development of diabetes, including rubella (German measles), mumps, Coxsackie virus, infectious hepatitis, infectious mononucleosis and cytomegalovirus (a form of herpes that usually afflicts those with impaired or immature immune systems). In animal studies, encephalomyocarditis (which causes inflammation of the heart muscle) and Venezuelan equine encephalitis (inflammation of the brain) also involve beta-cell destruction.

Some viruses may affect a child even before it is born: it has been estimated that an infant infected with rubella while in the womb has as high as a 40 percent chance of developing IDDM later in life.

Impaired Immune System: You learned in Chapter 1 that islet-cell antibodies were found in 90 percent of children first diagnosed with IDDM. It is still not known whether these antibodies were sent in as a reaction to some "foreign invader," such as the viruses described above, or are the result of a genetic defect that causes the body to produce substances that mistakenly attack its own pancreas. It may be either, depending on the case. But somewhere along the way, the immune system has faltered. People with IDDM also have higher risk of other autoimmune diseases, such as autoimmune thyroid disease, Addison's disease (a dysfunction of the adrenal gland), pernicious anemia, vitiligo (a skin disease resulting in loss of pigmentation), and myasthenia gravis (which is manifested by intermittent weakening of certain muscles).

Hormones: Because the typical age of onset for IDDM coincides with puberty, researchers suspect that it may be triggered by growth hormones, which would surely become more active around the time of increased physical development. An excess of growth hormone, released by the pituitary gland, is known to counteract insulin. Cortisol, an adrenal-gland hormone, has the same effect. The amount of hormone released can vary widely at certain times and under certain conditions, such as stress and infections, and it may be that a sustained increase can affect someone already predisposed to Type I diabetes. The same can be said for medications that contain hormones, such as cortisone or steroids. (For a more complete list of hormonal medications, see "Drugs" at the end of this chapter.)

Toxins and Other Chemicals: The rat poison Vacor has induced IDDM in people who ingested it by accident or in an attempt to commit suicide. (Banned in the U.S., the poison is still used in other parts of the world, such as Korea.) Alloxan and streptozocin (used in cancer therapy) directly damage beta cells. (For other chemicals and medications associated with diabetes, see "Drugs" at the end of this chapter.)

Diet: Because so few infants under nine months old have IDDM, a study was done to investigate whether breastfeeding has any effect on incidence. (Other research has indicated that breast-fed babies have fewer allergies as they grow older, because of milk-borne antibodies from the mother.) The results of this and a later study suggested that children with Type I were breast-fed for less time than their nondiabetic siblings or than the overall population. Such research has been limited, and another study failed to confirm these results, but it is possible that maternal antibodies also protect against IDDM.

A 1981 study related the parents' diet to a child's risk for diabetes. The reseachers noted that IDDM was high among Icelandic boys born in October, who would have been con-

ceived around Christmastime. Traditionally in Iceland during the holiday season, smoked or cured mutton is a
featured dish. This meat contains compounds similar to
streptozocin, a drug known to induce Type I diabetes.

Studies with mice have shown that changes in diet greatly
affect the rate of IDDM. But so far, scientists have not discovered how to apply this research to humans or which
specific components in food are responsible.

Stress: A severe trauma to the body—surgery, an injury,
burn, or infection—may also precede the development of
diabetes. Emotional stress, too, has been thought to precede
some cases of Type I diabetes. Stress can either interfere
with release of insulin from beta cells, or can stimulate the
release of hormones that counteract the effect of insulin on
lowering the blood sugar. Therefore, someone predisposed
to IDDM may be more vulnerable during stressful periods.

TYPE II RISK FACTORS

Age: The odds of getting Type II increase with age, as glucose tolerance naturally decreases as one grows older.
NIDDM usually occurs after age 40. (If the disease appears
before age 25, it is called MODY—maturity-onset diabetes
of the young.) If both of your parents had diabetes and you
live past 80, you will probably get NIDDM. One of the reasons that the incidence of the disease seems to be increasing
is that more and more people are living longer, thanks to
other advances in medicine.

Gender: Risk for NIDDM doesn't seem to be connected to
gender. Men are as likely as women to get the disease.

Race: Ethnic origins can point to a greater susceptibility to
Type II diabetes. The Pima Indians of Arizona and the na-
tives of Nauru, an island in the Central Pacific, claim the
highest rates of NIDDM: one in 12 Pimas and one in 36

islanders get diabetes after age 40. Rates are also high among other Native American tribes, Mexican Americans (many of whom also have Native American blood), and inhabitants of other Pacific Islands—Polynesia, Micronesia, Hawaii, and Samoa—and their descendants.

In the United States, blacks are more likely than whites to develop NIDDM. In fact, between 1966 and 1981, the numbers of blacks with Type II diabetes jumped 120 percent, while whites had only a 60 percent increase. More Hispanics—particularly those from Puerto Rico—who now live in America will develop NIDDM than those who remained in their native land.

Why some races are more susceptible to diabetes is open to debate. In this country, blacks, Native Americans, and Hispanics are not only more likely to have diabetes, they are also more likely to be poor, overweight, and less well educated—a deadly combination. They may not have access to information about proper nutrition needed to stay healthy and to control weight, or they may not be able to afford appropriate foods. (The cheapest products often undergo the most processing—which strips foods of vitamins, minerals, and fiber—and are the highest in salt, sugar, fat, and starch.) Native Americans restricted to reservations have lost the protection against diabetes that their traditional way of living and eating probably provided them.

Another theory proposes that particular populations may pass along a "thrifty gene." Throughout evolution, many races have had to live a "feast or famine" existence—with plenty to eat during some periods and virtual starvation at other times, depending on the growing season and other natural conditions. Over many generations, the body may have adjusted to this irregular eating pattern by changing the way it stored food for energy—actually becoming more efficient if food was limited. One proof of this theory was a 1979 study by Dr. Douglas Coleman of the Jackson Laboratory in Bar Harbor, Maine. When their food supply was cut off, mice bred to develop NIDDM lived 23 to 46 percent longer than normal mice. So it may be that, for people with this "thrifty gene," easy access to an abundance of food could lead the way to diabetes.

Socioeconomic Status: In nations where the economy is improving, higher income means higher rates of diabetes. In the United States, however, the poor have higher rates. This finding is probably related to eating habits and obesity: in less developed countries, the more affluent are turning to the Westernized "hamburger-and-fries" diet, while for lower-income Americans, inexpensive fast-food meals may be a staple and contribute to obesity.

Weight: There's no doubt that carrying extra pounds increases your chances of getting NIDDM if you have a family history of the disease. Not all overweight people get diabetes and not all diabetics are overweight, but 80 percent of those with diabetes are obese—meaning they're more than 20 percent over their ideal weight range (see chart at the end of this chapter). The longer you have been overweight, the greater your risk. In addition, the more overweight you are, the earlier diabetes will strike.

In one study of brothers and sisters of diabetics, the siblings who were obese were five times more likely to develop diabetes than those of normal weight. Unfortunately, obesity too seems to run in families, perhaps due to similar eating habits coupled with a genetic predisposition.

Where fat is distributed seems to be as significant as *how much.* If you tend to gain weight above the waist (the "apple-shaped" figure), you have a greater chance of diabetes than someone whose fat settles in hips and thighs (the pear shape). The higher the waist-to-hip ratio (see below), the greater the risk. Studies have shown this body shape also increases risk for heart disease and hypertension, both of which have been linked to diabetes.

To figure out your waist-to-hip ratio, you'll need a cloth tape measure—and a full-length mirror (or have someone else take your measurements). Without clothes or in underwear only, stand in front of the mirror with back straight, feet together, and stomach relaxed. Place the tape measure horizontally around your natural waist—the narrowest part of your torso, not necessarily over your navel. *Do not pull the tape tight against your skin.* Breathe out normally, then mark down the waist measurement within the nearest one-quarter inch. Next, place the tape around hips, at the widest point of the buttocks. Record this measurement to the nearest one-quarter inch. Divide the number for the waist into that for the hips. For instance, a waist measurement of 28¼ inches and a hip measurement of 37½ inches gives you a waist-to-hip ratio of 0.75. The healthiest ratio is *under* .80.

Inappropriate Diet: The high-fat, high-sugar, low-fiber meals and processed foods beloved by Americans have had their effect on diabetes around the world. As countries become more "Americanized," the cases of NIDDM seem to increase. Japanese who immigrate to Hawaii have double the diabetes rate of those still in Japan—even though both groups consume about the same number of calories. And the disease, once rare among Native Americans, has become rampant now that most have adopted a more modern lifestyle. Of course, the Western diet is also associated with weight gain, a major factor in NIDDM (see above). High blood-fat levels—often the result of eating too much saturated fat—and high uric acid levels—indicating an excess of protein—have been linked to diabetes. James Anderson, M.D., of the Veterans' Administration Hospital in Lexington, Kentucky, has worked to show that high-fiber diets can decrease blood sugar in diabetics, so a fiber-full menu may also work to keep glucose levels from ever becoming abnormal.

One point that should be made clear: sugar does not cause diabetes. What really happens is that someone who indulges a "sweet tooth" is also more apt to be overweight—and that condition is a trigger to NIDDM.

Inactivity: People who are not physically active add to their diabetes risk. Exercise improves glucose metabolism: trained athletes have lower blood-sugar levels and are more sensitive to insulin than nonathletes. In one study, women who were athletes in college were half as likely as the sedentary students to have diabetes in later years. On the other hand, prolonged bedrest is known to increase insulin resistance—and raise blood-sugar levels. Of course, avid exercisers are likely to use up more calories, and keep their weight within a healthy range.

Exercise also helps your body exchange fat for muscle. Studies of people with NIDDM who are not overweight have indicated that this group may be over*fat*—nonobese, but flabby from lack of activity. Couch potatoes, beware!

Stress: Stress—physical or mental—can influence blood-sugar levels in patients with diabetes, and may well trigger NIDDM in individuals with a genetic predisposition—and a family history—of the disease. It can also lead to uncontrolled eating and weight gain—thus adding greater risk of diabetes.

Pregnancy: Because of extra hormones released by the placenta, blood-glucose levels are always affected by pregnancy—even if you are not diagnosed as having gestational diabetes. Though studies have not yet proven it, it may be that the chance of developing diabetes increases with the number of pregnancies.

Gestational Diabetes: As was discussed in Chapter 1, having had impaired glucose tolerance while pregnant means you're more likely to develop NIDDM within the 15 years following delivery. Some studies have shown that the higher the mother's blood-glucose reading during this time or the higher the baby's weight at birth (over nine pounds), the greater the risk.

If your mother had diabetes while pregnant with you, your risk may increase. In a study of the Pima Indians, NIDDM occurred much more frequently among adolescents and young adults when the mother was diabetic during the pregnancy than among those whose mothers were not.

GESTATIONAL DIABETES

Gestational diabetes shares some of the risk factors of Type II diabetes but cannot really be considered in the same category. It usually appears without symptoms and is detected in routine tests given 24 to 28 weeks into the pregnancy. A woman with a family history of either Type I or Type II may be susceptible.

Age: You're more likely to become diabetic during pregnancy if you're over 30—probably because glucose tolerance naturally diminishes with age.

Weight: Like those with Type II, women who get gestational diabetes usually were overweight before becoming pregnant.

Impaired Glucose Intolerance: Your risk is increased if your blood-sugar levels have ever been even slightly elevated. Occasional sugar in the urine is also an indication of a future problem during pregnancy.

Previous Pregnancies: Did a previous pregnancy end in a stillbirth or have you delivered an unusually large or overweight infant (more than nine pounds)? These complications associated with maternal diabetes—even if you had not been diagnosed as having gestational diabetes at the time—are a predictor of diabetes in a later pregnancy.

DRUGS AND CHEMICALS

Certain medications can trigger diabetes or impair glucose tolerance by raising blood-sugar levels or affecting the pancreas's secretion of insulin. For instance, steroids—hormones that increase muscle mass—make the liver release glucose. Oral contraceptives that contain the synthetic estrogen *mestranol* impair glucose metabolism. Because oral diuretics cause you to lose water, you also lose potassium, which is necessary for the release of insulin. Drugs that stimulate the nervous system, such as epinephrine or amphetamines, can also stimulate the release of glycogen (stored glucose) and inhibit insulin production. Nicotinic acid (niacin) affects liver function and could worsen glucose intolerance or Type II diabetes.

Below is a more complete list of drugs associated with diabetes mellitus. (Specific brand names are given in parentheses.) Not enough is known about how each is implicated in diabetes and the impact it might have on those predisposed to the disease. However, if you have a family history of diabetes and are currently taking any of these medications, you should consult with your doctor. Only he or she can determine if your need for the drug outweighs the risk of diabetes.

Diuretics and Other High-Blood-Pressure Medications
Chlorthalidone (Hygroton, Combipres, Regroton)
Clonidine (Catapres, Combipres)
Diazoxide (Hyperstat, Proglycem)

Furosemide (Lasix)
Metalazone
Thiazides
Bumetanide
Clopamide
Clorexolone
Ethacrynic acid (Edecrin)

Hormonally active medications
Adrenocorticotropin (Acthar)
Glucagon
Glucocorticoids
Oral contraceptives
Somatotropin (growth hormone)
Thyroid hormone (thyrotoxic doses)
  Dextrothyroxine (Choloxin)
Calcitonin (Calcimar)
Medroxyprogesterone (Amen, Depo-Provera, Provera)
Prolactin

Mood-altering drugs
Chlorprothixene (Taractan)
Haloperidol (Haldol)
Lithium carbonate (Eskalith, Lithane)
Phenothiazines
  Chlorpromazine (Thorazine)
  Perphenazine (Trilafon, Etrafon, Triavil)
Clopenthixol
Tricyclic antidepressants
  Amitriptyline (Elavil, Endep, Etrafon, Triavil)
  Desipramine (Norpramin, Pertofrane)
  Doxepin (Adapin, Sinequan)
  Imipramine (Presamine, Tofranil, Imavata)
  Nortriptyline (Aventyl)
Marijuana

Catecholamines and other drugs that affect the nervous system

Diphenylhydantoin (Dilantin)
Epinephrine
Isoproterenol
Levodopa
Norepinephrine
Buphenine (Nylidrin)
Fenoterol
Propranolol (Inderal)

Analgesics, antipyretics (fever-reducers) and anti-inflammatories

Indomethacin (Indocin)
Acetaminophen*
Aspirin*
Morphine
*Only in very high doses

Cancer-therapy drugs

Alloxan
L-asparaginase
Streptozocin
Cyclophosphamide (Cytoxan)
Megestrol acetate (Megace)

Miscellaneous

Isoniazid (INH, Nydrazid, others)—treats tuberculosis
Nicotinic acid (niacin)—for high cholesterol; also available as a vitamin supplement
Cimetidine (Tagamet)—for ulcers
Edetic acid (EDTA)—used as an anticoagulant and to treat lead poisoning
Heparin—a heart medication that thins the blood
Mannoheptulose—derived from mannitol, a sugar alcohol
Nalidixic acid (NegGram)—treats urinary infections

Niridazole—for schistosomiasis, a parasitic infection

Pentamidine (Lomidine)—used to treat protozoal infections or to prevent pneumonia in those with impaired immune systems (such as AIDS patients)

Phenolphthalein (Ex-Lax)—relieves constipation

Thiabendazole—for parasitic worm infestations, such as trichinosis

Other chemicals that you may come in contact with at work or around the house can damage beta cells or affect blood-sugar levels. Talk to your doctor if you have a family history of diabetes and have been exposed to or have ingested any of the following.

Carbon disulfide—solvent for rubber, also used as an insecticide

Ethanol—ethyl alcohol, used as an antiseptic; also found in alcoholic beverages, though moderate drinking does not pose a risk (see Chapter 5)

Nickel chloride—used in nickel-plating cast zinc; the salts are sometimes found in gas masks because they can absorb other chemicals

Rodenticide (Vacor)—rat poison

Rate Your Risk

Are you at risk for diabetes? Could you already have it? Find out. The American Diabetes Association has prepared a simple test that helps you assess your own risk (for both types). Write in the points next to each statement that is true for you. If a statement is not true for you, put a zero. Then add up your total score.

1. I have been experiencing one or more of the following symptoms on a regular basis:
   - excessive thirst.. YES 3 _____
   - frequent urination .... YES 3 _____
   - extreme fatigue .... YES 1 _____

- unexplained weight loss............................ YES 3 _____
- blurry vision from time to time .... YES 1 _____
2. I am over 40 years old.................................... YES 1 _____
3. My weight is equal to or above that
listed in the chart below .... YES 2 _____
4. I am a woman who has had more than one baby
weighing over 9 pounds at birth..................... YES 2 _____
5. I am of Native American descent.................... YES 1 _____
6. I am of Hispanic or Black descent.................. YES 1 _____
7. I have a parent with diabetes.......................... YES 1 _____
8. I have a brother or sister with
diabetes.. YES 2 _____

                                                                       TOTAL _____

Weight Chart for Women

(shows 20% over ideal weights)

Height (without shoes)		Weight in Pounds (without clothing)
Feet	Inches	
4	9	113–127
4	10	116–131
4	11	120–134
5	0	124–138
5	1	127–142
5	2	131–146
5	3	134–151
5	4	139–157
5	5	144–162
5	6	149–167
5	7	154–172
5	8	158–176
5	9	163–181
5	10	168–186

Weight Chart for Men

(shows 20% over ideal weights)

Height (without shoes)		Weight in Pounds (without clothing)
Feet	Inches	
5	1	133–146
5	2	137–151
5	3	140–155
5	4	144–158
5	5	148–163
5	6	152–168
5	7	157–174
5	8	162–179
5	9	167–184
5	10	172–190
5	11	176–196
6	0	181–202
6	1	186–208
6	2	192–214
6	3	198–220

This chart shows a range: e.g. 113 is 20% overweight for a small-boned woman at 4′9″; 127 is for a larger frame.

Scoring

3 to 5 Points: If you scored 3 to 5 points you probably are at low risk for diabetes. But don't just forget about it—

especially if you're over 40, overweight, or of Black, Hispanic or Native American Indian descent.

What to do about it: Be sure you know the symptoms of diabetes (turn to the next chapter). If you experience any of these symptoms, contact your doctor for further testing.

Over 5 Points: If you scored over 5 points, you may be at high risk for diabetes. You may even already have diabetes.

What to do about it: See your doctor promptly. Find out if you have diabetes. Even if you don't have diabetes, know the symptoms [turn to the next chapter]. If you experience any of them in the future, you should see your doctor immediately.

Please note: This test is meant to educate and make you aware of the serious risks of diabetes. Only a medical doctor can determine if you do have diabetes. The American Diabetes Association also urges all pregnant women to be tested for diabetes between the 24th and 28th weeks of pregnancy.

CHAPTER

3

Signs and Symptoms

B Y now, you have determined how much at risk you and your family are for diabetes. It is hoped that you will begin, with the help of the later chapters in this book, to alter those factors you can change.

But in your determination to prevent diabetes, do not ignore the very real possibility that problems may still lie ahead for you or your loved ones. Just as heredity does not give you a 100 percent guarantee of developing diabetes, changes made at this point in your life are not a 100 percent guarantee that the disorder will not surface, though in a milder form than you might otherwise have suffered. If you have a history of the disease in your family, you should be especially alert to the range of signs and symptoms that may signal impending diabetes or may be the first evidence of the disorder.

Right now, about 14 million people in the United States have diabetes. But only half of these people know that they have it. The rest may go for years without being diagnosed, because the symptoms can be subtle or they can appear to be a different problem altogether. In the meantime, the disease may be upsetting other systems in the body.

Any symptoms should be brought to your doctor's attention immediately. He or she can perform tests to rule out or confirm the presence of diabetes. The earlier the diagnosis, the better your chances of controlling the illness and heading off its most serious consequences.

And the consequences of diabetes are serious indeed. Blindness, heart disease, kidney failure, and nerve damage have all been linked to diabetes that has gone undiagnosed or is poorly controlled for too long. As the disease progresses, slowed blood flow and nerve loss, most often in the feet and legs, may lead to gangrene (dead tissue), and the foot or leg may have to be amputated. Each year more than 150,000 persons die from diabetes and its complications—the seventh leading cause of death in the United States.

These statistics may frighten you—and they should. But what is more unsettling is that many of these conditions could have been avoided, or certainly been less severe, if people aware of their risk had done all that they could toward safeguarding their health. You can help your own efforts by familiarizing yourself and your family with the early warnings and symptoms of diabetes.

EARLY WARNINGS

Several health problems may show themselves even before blood glucose reaches the level where it can be diagnosed as diabetes. If you have a family history of diabetes and experience any one of these problems, it could be a precursor to the disorder and should be thoroughly checked out with your doctor.

Skin: All blood vessels are affected by diabetes, including those that nourish the skin. When the nutrients, oxygen, and moisture that blood normally brings to the body's surface are cut off or diminished in some way, the skin's texture or appearance may change. Skin may be unusually dry or it may be itchy, particularly in genital and anal areas. You may notice a "shin spot"—a brown, scaly patch about the size of a dime on the front of the lower leg. It may have begun as an accidental bump to the shin, but why the spot appears is not certain. It happens more often to men than women.

Skin infections may become common. Boils (small, painful lumps) or carbuncles (clusters of boils or abscesses), both caused by bacteria, may appear anywhere on the body, often on the back of the neck. These infections may recur and be difficult to get rid of. In fact, any wound on the skin that takes longer to heal may be a warning of current or future diabetes.

Be aware of persistent fungal infections, especially on the feet. While athlete's foot is common to everyone, in those with a family history of diabetes it may have more significance. The same is true for women who have candidiasis, also known as yeast infection, which causes vaginal itching and a whitish discharge. (Since yeasts feed on sugar, excess glucose in the system presents the perfect environment for this gynecological problem.) In general, the conditions of diabetes can reduce the body's ability to fight any infection.

Complications in Pregnancy: As mentioned in the previous chapter, elevated blood sugar during pregnancy, or gestational diabetes, can be a warning of diabetes to come. Other problems with childbirth—a premature or difficult delivery, frequent miscarriages, toxemia (bacterial blood poisoning), and the birth of a baby weighing more than nine pounds—may also precede a diagnosis of diabetes. In addition, diabetes in the mother may interfere with fetal development, resulting in birth defects (such as abnormal communications between the chambers of the heart).

Hypoglycemia: *Low* blood sugar may also herald early or mild Type II diabetes—it could indicate a problem with how the body is producing and using insulin. (Of course, hypoglycemia is also a concern for people already being treated for Type I diabetes; it occurs if they inject too much insulin or attempt vigorous exercise without eating enough to balance the need for extra energy.) Hypoglycemia usually occurs about three to four hours after a meal, starting with feelings of hunger, nervousness, trembling, headache, weakness, or confusion. The symptoms are usually relieved by eating; if not, you may feel faint or lose consciousness at these times.

Arterial Disease: There are several mechanisms by which diabetes affects the heart, arteries, and all blood vessels—the cardiovascular system. Someone with heart disease or arteriosclerosis (hardening of the arteries) at an uncommonly young age (before menopause in women) may have undiagnosed diabetes.

Diabetic Complications: Sometimes, the dire consequences of long-time diabetes can surface even before symptoms of elevated blood sugar are evident. For instance, diabetic retinopathy is an eye disorder brought on by changes in the blood vessels due to diabetes; the tiny vessels of the retina (the light-sensitive membrane that lines the eyeball) may break or leak blood inside the eye. Neuropathy, damage to nerves, may be noticed as numbness or tingling in the feet or legs. Albumin, a form of protein, may show up in the urine because the kidney has been impaired by diabetic conditions. Impotence can also be a problem for men, if damage to nerves or blood vessels has already begun. Though other disorders can cause these problems too, having any one of these conditions should alert you to the possibility of diabetes in the future.

TYPE I SYMPTOMS

The symptoms associated with the insulin-dependent form of diabetes are so distinct that they rarely leave any doubt of the diagnosis. Unfortunately, their onset is often so rapid that the patient has little warning—perhaps a few days or weeks—even though the destruction of beta cells may have begun years before. The start of Type I may be more gradual in older persons. However, IDDM usually strikes the young, and it's easy to dismiss some of the symptoms as flu or another childhood ailment. It's up to parents who know that diabetes runs in the family to be aware of these signs, and to contact their doctor if they notice any physical or behavioral changes in their children.

Polyuria: As you'll remember from Chapter 1, urinating frequently and in large amounts is a classic symptom of diabetes, as the body rushes fluids through the kidney to dilute the high levels of sugar in the urine. Because of this, a child who no longer wets the bed may resume having this problem when IDDM begins.

Polydipsia: An unusual thirst is a natural result of too frequent urination: the body is signaling for lost fluids to be replaced. Dehydration will eventually occur if the condition is not caught early.

Polyphagia: This feeling of extreme hunger stems from the body's belief that it is starving because glucose is not reaching its cells to provide desperately needed energy.

Rapid Weight Loss: Unlike the majority of Type II patients, most of those who eventually get Type I are at or below their ideal weight. When IDDM begins, they may suddenly lose more weight—as much as 15 pounds in a week—even though they may be eating more than enough and have a good appetite. The lack of insulin means that calories, in the form of glucose, are being sent out through the urine, and the body is beginning to burn fat reserves.

Weakness: Since muscle cells are not receiving their usual fuel, energy flags. Of course, fatigue can have many causes, which is why diabetes can go unrecognized for so long. Be concerned if a once active child seems tired, drowsy, or listless for no apparent reason. Some children may also complain of stomach, leg, or chest pains, or have difficulty breathing.

Irritability: In youngsters, crankiness, confusion or excessive crying may warn of impending illness. A child may seem to be inattentive or may not be doing as well in school as before.

Nausea and/or Vomiting: These symptoms may precede ketoacidosis, as poisonous ketone acids build up in the blood when the body must resort to burning fat deposits for energy.

Blurred Vision: Excess glucose may be seeping into the eye, changing the shape of the lens. Difficulty in focusing or changes in eyesight from one day to the next—such as from nearsighted to normal vision—are other visual cues for possible diabetes.

Slowed Growth: If cells are not being nourished sufficiently, as happens with IDDM, children may not develop as they should. A youngster inclined towards diabetes may be smaller than average for his or her age.

TYPE II SYMPTOMS

Non-insulin-dependent diabetes can creep along unnoticed for years. Symptoms may appear gradually, becoming more intense or frequent with age. By then, however, the damage to other systems of the body—eyes, blood vessels, nerves— may have already started.

Any of Type I Warning Signs: Of course, these symptoms may be more subtle in those with Type II. You should also be aware that even overweight people—who make up the majority of those with NIDDM—may have a sudden, unexplained weight loss at first.

Blurred Vision or Other Changes in Eyesight: This may be the result of glucose affecting the lens or the signs of retinopathy, as explained in "Early Warnings." Beginning damage to the nerves that move the eye muscles might also be the cause of occasional blurry or double vision.

Tingling or Numbness in Legs, Feet, or Fingers: Or you may have a burning sensation or heightened sensitivity in these extremities or on other spots on your skin. Symptoms, such as leg cramps, may appear or worsen only at night. Again, these may be signs that circulation is poor or that nerve damage is already progressing.

Frequent Infections: Diabetes weakens the body's defenses against invasions of bacteria. Infections of the gums, urinary tract, or skin that keep recurring or take a long time to clear up show that the disease may have begun interfering with the immune system.

Itching of Skin or Genitals: This may be the result of an underlying infection or dehydration, a common by-product of diabetes.

Slow Healing of Cuts and Bruises: Because diabetes affects how the nutrients obtained from food are used by cells, the body may have difficulty repairing damaged tissue. Diabetes also thickens blood vessels, slowing circulation and preventing wounds from receiving, through the blood, these needed nutrients and oxygen.

Drowsiness: Again, feeling tired often and for too long means energy is not getting to cells. This is a common symptom, often overlooked.

Unfortunately, too many of these symptoms can be overlooked or blamed on other conditions. The only way to be sure of their connection to diabetes is to see your doctor, who will perform some simple tests to determine your glucose levels. The next chapter will describe these tests and how they may help you and your family even *before* diabetes takes hold.

CHAPTER

4

The Importance of
Early Detection

HAVE you experienced any of the signs of diabetes discussed in the preceding chapter? If you haven't, you may feel much less worried about the immediate danger of diabetes. If you have, perhaps the symptom did not seem alarming enough to push you to the next step—seeing your doctor for a diabetes screening. Unfortunately, you can't rely on symptoms alone to alert you to potential problems.

Diabetes is not always obvious. In Type I, signs usually do not appear until approximately 90 percent of the beta cells have already been destroyed. In Type II, symptoms may never be noticeable. Meanwhile, the disease is insidiously interfering with the major systems of the body.

Some of the consequences of undiscovered or untreated diabetes were touched on in Chapter 3. Most are related to how the disease chemically affects the blood vessels—from the tiny capillaries in the eyes and kidneys to the main arteries leading to the heart, brain, and legs. The blood they carry nourishes and brings oxygen to all tissues. But diabetes can restrict this blood flow by thickening or weakening vessel walls. The following conditions can result:

Blindness: In the United States, the leading cause of vision loss among 20- to 74-year-olds is diabetic retinopathy—when vessels in the retina rupture or hemorrhage into the eye. Luckily, many cases of retinopathy can now be helped with a newly perfected laser treatment called photocoagulation. However, if diabetes goes untreated, retinopathy may progress too, increasing the risk of permanent visual impairment.

Diabetics are also prone to other visual problems: 12 percent have cataracts (clouding of the lens) and 11 percent report glaucoma (the buildup of pressure from fluid in the eye). For both conditions, these figures are two to three times that found in the general population.

Kidney Disease: About 35 percent of Type I diabetics, and perhaps the same number of those with Type II, have this condition, called nephropathy. Thickened blood vessels in the kidneys interfere with the organs' ability to filter protein and to eliminate bodily wastes: useful protein is lost, while toxic waste products accumulate in the blood. The kidneys are also harmed by the recurring urinary-tract infections common to diabetes. Eventually, the kidneys may stop functioning entirely, and dialysis or a transplant may be necessary.

Neuropathy: Nerve cells are highly sensitive to the body's chemical changes, and diabetes is considered the most common cause of nerve damage in Western countries. Estimates vary widely, but it is thought that more than 40 percent of those with diabetes will eventually suffer nerve impairment. This can affect sensation in the legs, feet, hands, and joints. It also interferes with control of digestive, urinary, and sexual functions, bringing on episodes of diarrhea, bladder problems, or impotence.

Vascular Disease: Having diabetes doubles a person's risk of dying from heart disease. Twice as many people with diabetes as without will have some form of heart trouble. When blood vessels to the brain are affected, diabetics are two to six times more likely to suffer a stroke; cerebrovascular diseases are apparent in one-fourth of the deaths due to diabetes.

When blood circulation is obstructed, blood pressure rises—as is the case for half of those with diabetes. Having hypertension adds to your risk of other complications—kidney disease, retinopathy, heart disease, and stroke.

Vascular disease and other diabetic complications may contribute—together or separately is not certain—toward the development of gangrene. Nerve damage can make feet insensitive to injury. Infection, which a diabetes-weakened body has difficulty fighting, may set in. Poor circulation may prevent the infection or injury from healing: the decreased blood flow keeps oxygen and nutrients, as well as antibiotics, from reaching the infected area. Eventually, normal tissue deteriorates and dies; toes or a foot may have to be amputated. Diabetes is present in at least 50 percent of people who need amputations for reasons other than direct physical injury to the limb.

For those whose diabetes has been diagnosed and is under control, the horrific complications associated with the disease are relatively uncommon. Early diagnosis is crucial, so that necessary treatment can begin and halt the progression of these other problems. If you have a family history of diabetes, you already are at risk and should meet with your doctor so he or she can determine your current medical condition and perform the standard screening and diagnostic tests, which are described below.

In addition to aiding in early detection of diabetes, these tests may indicate your future risk even if the results are negative. It must be noted that the tests currently in use

may not disclose every case of diabetes, or may indicate the
disease when it may not be present. No single test is 100 percent accurate or comprehensively sensitive, because so many
variables can affect the outcome. Some examples follow.

General Health: Certain chronic illnesses, such as kidney
or liver disease, can affect test outcome. If you have an acute
illness, like an infection or the flu, you probably shouldn't
be tested until several months after the condition has
cleared up. Someone suffering from malnutrition or under
emotional stress should also wait until the problem is alleviated. For some people even the stress or fear of the testing itself can elevate blood glucose for a while.

Age: We know that glucose tolerance diminishes as we age.
Unfortunately, it's not known whether this indicates a normal bodily change unrelated to diabetes or if it shows a true
increase in symptom-free diabetes. This makes it difficult
to reliably apply the same criteria for glucose levels to all
age groups.

Medications: Drugs that alter or affect blood sugar are listed
at the end of Chapter 2. In addition, some of these medications can lower glucose levels: monoamine oxidase inhib-
itors (antidepressants also known as MAOs), beta blockers
(used for high blood pressure and heart arrhythmia), sul-
fonamides (for treating urinary-tract and other infections),
phenylbutazone and other pyrazolone derivatives (for inflammation such as arthritis), bishydroxycoumarin (to prevent blood clotting), and alcohol. Anyone using any of these
chemicals may give a false reading on a glucose tolerance
test. Doctors usually have patients discontinue medications
at least three days prior to testing, if possible.

Diet: What is ingested in the week before testing can interfere with glucose levels. For instance, drinking coffee or

smoking can alter metabolism; neither is allowed before or during the test. In addition, patients often attempt to diet just before seeing their doctors, afraid they'll be reprimanded about their weight. However, if you restrict food, particularly carbohydrates, for several days preceding a diagnostic test, that can mean a false positive for diabetes. This is also true for anyone who has anorexia or other eating disorders.

Physical Activity: Too much or too little activity prior to a test can influence the results. This precludes from testing anyone who is unable to walk or has been bedridden for three days or more. Physicians also discourage excessive exercise beforehand.

Generally, doctors are not willing to perform screening tests for diabetes without cause to suspect the disorder, believing that an incorrect diagnosis may do more psychological harm than physical good. Random testing of the general population with glucose-tolerance tests is frowned upon. However, once-a-year screening is encouraged for individuals who are considered to be in any one of these high-risk groups:

- persons who have a strong family history of diabetes;
- those who are 20 percent over their ideal weight;
- women who have had a stillbirth or a baby over 9 pounds, or had toxemia or glycosuria during pregnancy;
- those with a history of recurrent skin, urinary-tract, or genital infections.

All pregnant women, regardless of other factors, should be tested in the seventh month of pregnancy.

URINE TESTING

Most of us are familiar with the testing of urine for sugar: during a checkup at the gynecologist or an annual physical, it's routine to be asked to provide a urine sample. This may lead you to believe that you are already being regularly checked for diabetes. Certainly a positive result for sugar on a urinalysis should alert your doctor to look further into the problem. But the truth is that a urinalysis is not sufficient to discover diabetes, and it is not the first choice for screening someone with a likelihood of developing the disease.

Sugar in the urine could have a number of causes other than diabetes. In children, for instance, the presence of sugar in the urine more often indicates "renal glycosuria." The kidneys of a still-developing child may not be able to filter enough useful glucose before losing it to elimination, so the sugar winds up in the urine. Also, pregnant women may show increased sugar in the urine, and nursing mothers may be excreting lactose (milk sugar). In these cases, only a blood-glucose test will document normal levels.

You could have a negative result on a urinalysis and still have diabetes. Each of us has a "renal threshold"—the limit to how much glucose our kidneys can recover. This threshold may be higher for some people—usually older adults—than for others. By the time sugar appears in their urine, diabetes may have been present for quite some time.

More often, urine testing is used by those who already have diabetes and perform a self-test to evaluate their control. But even then, the amount of sugar in the urine may not reflect the amount of sugar in the blood *at that moment*—the urinalysis frequently shows what blood-glucose levels were like several hours earlier. For people with diabetes, a urine sample is the only way to test for ketones—an early warning sign that the disease may be out of control due to the total lack of insulin. But for those being screened for diabetes, the urinalysis cannot be used to make a definitive diagnosis.

SCREENING TESTS

In diabetes testing, glucose levels are given either as mg/
dL (milligrams per deciliter) or as mg% (milligrams percent). For example, normal glucose levels are between 60
and 120 mg/dl or 60 and 120 mg%—meaning that each 100
cubic centimeters (cc) of blood contains between 60 and 120
milligrams of glucose.

Blood-sugar levels fluctuate, depending on the time of day
and when food was last eaten. For instance, glucose tolerance usually decreases toward the afternoon and for five to
10 hours after a meal. The level rises for about an hour after
eating, then drops rapidly—and within two to three hours
may be back down to the level it was before breakfast. Because of these hourly changes, most tests are performed at
specific times and with strict guidelines regarding food consumption.

Random Blood-Sugar Level

For this screening, a blood sample can be drawn at any time
of day if food or drink has been taken within three hours
of testing. When the obvious signs of diabetes (polyuria,
polydipsia, polyphagia, weight loss, fatigue, blurred vision,
ketones in urine) are present, a glucose reading of 200 mg/
dl or higher indicates a diagnosis of diabetes in children or
nonpregnant adults of any age.

Fasting Blood Sugar

This simple blood test is most often used to screen for diabetes, though it is less sensitive than an oral glucose tolerance test (described below). A blood sample is drawn in
the morning before any food has been eaten. At this time,
average blood-glucose levels range between 60 and 100 mg/
dl; a normal reading should be below 115 mg/dl. If it is 140
mg/dl or above, a second testing is usually done to confirm
the elevated glucose level. If both are high, diabetes is the

diagnosis for a nonpregnant adult. For children, a normal level is under 130 mg/dl; if the level is higher than that and if the child shows no classic signs of diabetes, oral glucose-tolerance tests are usually performed on two occasions to ensure a correct diagnosis. In pregnant women, a fasting blood-glucose level of 105 mg/dl or more indicates the need for further testing of glucose tolerance.

For adults, a glucose level between 105 and 140 mg/dl may signal impaired glucose tolerance and requires an oral glucose-tolerance test to rule out diabetes. Though falling within this range does signify a higher than normal risk for later diabetes, it should not be considered a final diagnosis. Your physician should keep an eye on your condition with regular follow-up testing. You'll probably also be advised to lose weight, if you are obese, or to otherwise modify your life-style to eliminate risks to your cardiovascular system. This might include cutting down on fats and cholesterol, quitting smoking, adding fiber to your diet, and increasing exercise.

Even if fasting blood-sugar levels are found to be normal, diabetes cannot be totally ruled out. Sometimes blood sugar can be fine during fasting, but elevate abnormally after eating. Your doctor will decide whether you need further diagnostic testing.

Oral Glucose Load for Gestational Diabetes

If you are pregnant, you will undergo regular fasting blood-glucose tests during scheduled prenatal visits to your doctor. However, even several episodes of testing may not catch a case of gestational diabetes. If the condition has not been detected before the 24th to 28th week, a test similar to the oral glucose-tolerance test (described below) will be performed. You will be given a 50-gram dose of glucose no matter what time of day or when you had your last meal. A blood sample is taken one hour later. A positive result— 140 mg/dl or more—requires an oral glucose-tolerance test.

DIAGNOSTIC TESTS

When the obvious symptoms of diabetes are absent, a fasting blood-sugar test is often all that's necessary to decide or dismiss a suspicion of the disease. However, a more sensitive diagnostic test may be called for in certain circumstances, such as:

- when fasting blood-glucose values are borderline or are abnormal but not high enough to suggest diabetes.
- if the results of screening tests are positive for diabetes.
- if the patient has a family history of MODY.
- when testing for gestational diabetes.
- if the patient is experiencing any of the obvious symptoms of diabetes mellitus—frequent urination, extreme hunger or thirst, weight loss.
- if someone does not have any symptoms but is obese and has a strong family history of diabetes.
- for individuals with otherwise unexplained nerve damage, retinopathy, heart or blood-vessel disease, kidney malfunction—particularly if the person is less than 50 years old.
- for those with abnormal glucose levels or sugar in the urine discovered while being treated for other conditions (for instance, heart or vascular disease), during surgery or emotional stress, or while taking steroids.

Oral Glucose-Tolerance Test

This procedure measures the body's response to receiving sudden large amounts of glucose. It's the most accurate way to eliminate any doubt of diabetes.

The person being tested is usually instructed to eat plenty of carbohydrates for the three to five days beforehand—about 200 grams per day. One ounce of bread, or a half cup of cereal, grains, pasta, or fruit each contains about 15 grams of carbohydrate; one cup of milk has 12; a half cup of any vegetable, 5. That translates into about 14 to 15 servings daily of any combination of starchy foods. (For more about serving sizes, turn to the Exchange Lists in Chapter 5.) A pre-test diet under 150 grams of carbohydrates could trigger an abnormal reaction to glucose: a low-carbohydrate diet depletes the liver of glycogen stores; the liver becomes sluggish and then, when bombarded with glucose during the test, cannot gather up the excess quickly enough. That extra glucose in the blood might be measured as diabetes, though it is not truly present.

For the 10 to 14 hours just prior to testing, no food or drink except water is allowed . The morning of the test, the physician will first draw a blood sample to measure fasting blood-glucose levels. Next, the patient drinks a glucose solution, usually 300 milliliters of fruit- or cola-flavored water containing a specific amount of glucose—75 grams for nonpregnant adults and 100 grams for pregnant women; children are given 1.75 grams per kilogram of their ideal body weight (calculated by height and age), up to 75 grams. A blood sample is then taken every 30 minutes for two hours (nonpregnant adults or children) or every hour for three hours (pregnant women).

In nonpregnant adults, a diagnosis of diabetes is reached if high fasting glucose levels are found during at least two oral glucose-tolerance tests. (See chart on page 57.) Some adjustment for age may be made for older adults, allowing an extra 10 mg/dl (at the two-hour interval) for each decade over 50 years old.

The criteria are different for pregnant women and children (see chart). During pregnancy, glucose levels too low to show diabetes may still be harmful to the fetus. Also, in any normal pregnancy, fasting blood sugar tends to drop more than usual, and levels tend to climb quickly once glucose is ingested. Children's readings are generally lower than those of adults on glucose-tolerance tests.

The chart at right compares normal test results with readings that indicate diabetes or impaired glucose tolerance.

Intravenous Glucose-Tolerance Test

Not a usual procedure, this method would be administered if you had gastrointestinal problems or another condition that interferes with normal absorption of glucose. It is also used sometimes as a research procedure. It is similar to the oral glucose-tolerance test, except that a smaller amount of glucose (about 25 grams) is given intravenously, rather than taken by mouth. This test is also quicker (values are taken within an hour) and less likely to cause nausea.

Oral Cortisone- or Steroid-Glucose-Tolerance Test

This method is rarely used outside of research situations, but may eventually be helpful in detecting potential diabetes in relatives of diabetics. Reports show that giving a dose of cortisone or another steroid just before an oral glucose-tolerance test points out a defect in carbohydrate metabolism in some people who have otherwise normal glucose levels. The hormone acts, in effect, like pregnancy—chemically stressing glucose tolerance. The standard values on this test are slightly higher than on the regular oral glucose-tolerance test.

TESTS IN THE WORKS

Research is also under way to develop tests that will determine who is liable to get diabetes, years before glucose levels are abnormal enough to be picked up with current testing methods. The challenge then becomes how to intervene to keep diabetes from surfacing.

Antibody Screening

Though not yet widely available, a few tests already exist that offer some hope to those who fear they or their children may inherit Type I diabetes. Physicians are now able to test

Results of Glucose-Tolerance Tests

Diagnosis	Nonpregnant Adult	Child	Pregnant Woman
Normal			
Fasting	under 115	under 130	under 105
30, 60, or 90 minutes after glucose	under 200	—	under 150
2 hours after glucose	under 140	under 140	—
Impaired Glucose Tolerance			
Fasting	under 140	under 140 **plus**	—
30, 60 or 90 minutes after glucose	200 or over	—	—
2 hours after glucose	140 to 200	over 140	—
Diabetes Mellitus			
Two or more fasting samples	over 140 **or**	140 or over **plus**	—
30, 60 or 90 minutes after glucose	over 200 **plus**	200 or over **plus**	—
2 hours after glucose	over 200	200 or over	—
3 hours after glucose	—	—	—
Gestational Diabetes (any two intervals)			
Two or more fasting samples	—	—	105 or over
30, 60 or 90 minutes after glucose	—	—	190 or over
2 hours after glucose	—	—	165 or over
3 hours after glucose	—	—	145 or over

blood samples for levels of ICAs—the islet-cell antibodies that were discussed in Chapter 1. These antibodies may begin circulating as much as 10 years before the onset of IDDM, indicating that the attack on the beta cells has already started.

It is estimated that two to three percent of first-degree relatives—offspring, brothers and sisters, mother and father—of someone with IDDM will test positive. Unfortunately, the screening may not catch about 30 percent of those family members headed for IDDM.

While a negative result on the test may put many people's minds at rest, a positive reading presents many problems. First of all, it does not mean that diabetes will ever develop—it just indicates an increased risk. More important, knowing that the antibodies exist is not enough—the physician must have a way of stopping them from acting. Currently, no surefire treatment is available.

Some ongoing experiments are having encouraging results. One study at the University of Florida is using azathioprine, an immunosuppressant drug, to try to block the production of antibodies. (Immunosuppressants are often used in transplant therapy, to keep the body from rejecting the "foreign" organ.) A 21-year-old woman susceptible to Type I has not developed any symptoms while taking the drug daily for the past five years. At the Joslin Diabetes Center in Boston, insulin alone has been administered daily to a group of individuals identified as "prediabetic"; the center reports that their first phase insulin release—the body's earliest response to insulin release—"has moved from the near-diabetic range into the normal range."

But until effective treatments are developed, the discovery of antibodies could also inflict psychological damage on the individual. There are fears that this stress may contribute to the development of IDDM. As it is, antibody testing is being limited to those known already to be at greater risk—first-degree relatives of Type I patients. If results are pos-

itive, more tests are given to determine how far beta-cell
destruction has gone, if at all, and follow-up tests are performed regularly.

Testing is also possible for insulin autoantibodies (IAAs),
which attach to insulin in the blood. They're found in 28 to
50 percent of people newly diagnosed with Type I. If a person has both IAAs and ICAs, the risk of developing diabetes
in the future would be greater than for having either type
of antibody alone.

An even better marker may be antibodies directed against
64K—an antigen protein on the surface of beta cells. Tests
have detected 64K antibodies in 71 to 88 percent of Type I
patients, up to eight years before onset. As yet, though,
screening for 64K antibodies is time-consuming and costly.

Massimo Trucco and colleagues at the University of Pittsburgh School of Medicine have developed a test that may
predict Type I before any beta-cell destruction has begun.
DNA from white blood cells is analyzed for a genetic flaw:
the absence of aspartic acid at position 57 of the HLA-DQ
beta chain (discussed in Chapter 1). The test is based on
recent research suggesting that this amino acid protects
against diabetes by keeping antibodies from attaching to
beta cells. Persons without aspartic acid at this specific location are thought to be 107 times more likely to develop
IDDM. The test's accuracy and practicality have yet to be
confirmed.

Insulin Levels

Researchers have noticed that healthy patients and those
with mild diabetes differ in the amount of insulin present
in the bloodstream before and after glucose is given in
glucose-tolerance tests. Though this variation is not used
to diagnose diabetes, decreased levels of insulin following
a glucose challenge would indicate a greater risk for the
disease. This risk is increased if a person has this decreased
insulin response and also tests positive for ICAs.

Glycosylation

Right now, doctors can see how well a patient with diabetes is controlling blood sugar, even over several weeks, by measuring his or her percentage of glycosylated hemoglobin, also called glycohemoglobin, glycated hemoglobin, or HgbA1C. A substance in the red blood cells, hemoglobin carries oxygen to other cells. Glycosylation occurs during periods of high blood-sugar levels, when some glucose attaches to the hemoglobin and remains there for the life of the red blood cell containing hemoglobin—about 120 days. Because of this process, testing can determine the average blood-sugar levels for the one to two months prior to the test. Depending on the results, adjustments can be made in the patient's diabetes treatment. In general, diabetic patients with many complications exhibit much higher HgbA1C levels than patients without complications.

Other types of cells besides hemoglobin are also subject to glycosylation. Recently tests have been devised that measure by-products of an advanced stage of glycosylation in proteins in the kidneys, blood vessels, and other tissues. The presence of these AGEs (advanced glycosylation end products) in the blood can warn that diabetic complications have begun, requiring treatment to prevent them from progressing further.

Electron Microscope

Already, studies have used this highly sensitive microscope to examine blood vessel walls for thickening caused by diabetes. However, these membranes can be obtained only from certain tissues (such as in muscle, skin, and kidneys) and the composition of these tissues themselves are so different that it's impractical to use this test to diagnose diabetes. Still, the search is on to try to detect the earliest changes in tissue with the electron microscope, so as to predict who may be headed for diabetes.

Receptors

In Type II diabetes, glucagon as well as insulin is less able to attach to cells. Georgetown University researchers discovered that nine out of 10 offspring of persons with diabetes had fewer glucagon receptors than normal; though they had no symptoms of disease, their ability to bind this hormone was only about one-third that of those with no family history of diabetes. So far, testing for receptors is too complex for practical application; also the condition can be detected about the same time as glycosylated hemoglobin—a measurement that can be more easily obtained.

SELF-TESTING

You've probably noticed them in your local pharmacy: kits for testing one's own glucose levels. Inside are chemically treated strips for testing a finger-pricked blood sample or for measuring sugar or ketones in urine. Digitized meters that give off more precise readings are also available at drugstore counters. Soon, bloodless devices will be available which can measure blood glucose levels of the finger using a near-infra-red spectroscopy method.

People who have diabetes and are under treatment by a doctor often monitor their own glucose levels—occasionally or frequently, depending on the severity of the disease. This not only helps the physician keep track of an individual's progress, but it also gives the patient more control and responsibility for her or his condition. That may seem like a burden, but in reality it helps a person with diabetes feel like a part of the team that is managing his or her health.

Some people with Type I diabetes have used store-bought kits to test their children for IDDM. The concern is that the person should know how to use the test and evaluate the results properly. Someone who is not already under a doctor's care for diabetes should not attempt to self-test without consulting a physician.

Another consideration is the psychological effect of testing yourself or another. Certainly, if the test is performed periodically on a child, the youngster may experience anxiety about becoming sick. Trying to diagnose a disease to which you or your family may or may not be susceptible can be an unhealthy preoccupation. In turn, the stress could theoretically add to your risk of developing the disease!

Finally, you should be aware that testing materials can be expensive. Unless your doctor recommends using these kits, you probably will not be compensated for the cost by your health-insurance carrier—therefore adding financial strain to your worries.

If you want to feel in control of your diabetic destiny, the best and surest approach is to lower your risk. The next chapters tell you how.

CHAPTER

5

Beating the Odds
Through Diet

IF someone in your family already has diabetes, you know
that diet is the most essential component of her or his
treatment. For many Type II patients, weight loss may be
enough to alleviate symptoms. Does that mean that, as an
at-risk relative, you have to follow some rigid "diabetic diet"
even before you have any signs of disease?

No, because you don't need to concern yourself with the
timing and frequency of meals, or the specifics of keeping
blood-glucose levels steady. But those with diabetes do learn
about good nutrition—and so should you. For them, the
consequences of not following a healthy eating plan are
more immediate—unstable blood-glucose levels, weakness,
and the onset of complications. For you, the consequences—
diabetes or another health problem—may appear much
later. In truth, the basics of a "diabetic diet" are not unique
to the treatment of diabetes; they can protect you from hypertension, heart disease, cancer, and a variety of other ills.
These basic diet guidelines are the prescription for anyone
who wants to enjoy a longer, healthier life.

Perhaps when you hear the word *diet,* you think *depri-
vation,* sure that it means you won't ever be able to enjoy
the foods you like. If you're overweight, you may also think

starvation, expecting that a strict reduction of food is the only way to slim down.

Unfortunately, both these "myth-definitions" have been perpetuated by manufacturers of products that promise quick slimming or instant good health—without promising that they will satisfy your appetite, taste good, or fit into your life-style. These special drinks, powders, and pills, books that promote "magic" (and unappetizing) menus for weight loss or longevity, and even vitamin supplements— which imply that you can bypass food and still get all the nutrients you need—don't, and can't, promise permanent or even long-lasting results. They give the word *diet* a bad name.

First and foremost, *diet* means "regular nourishment." We all need to take in carbohydrates, proteins, and fats to meet our daily energy requirements. From these fuels come the vitamins, minerals, and other compounds that maintain mental and physical functioning, and the growth and repair of cells. The best source is food, real food, of all kinds.

Of course, the body has use for only certain amounts of fuel each day. The excess of some nutrients may be excreted (for instance, water-soluble vitamins, such as vitamin C, are passed through the urine); the rest is stored as fat. If too much is stored without the possibility of its being used in the near future, the body registers a weight gain.

Avoiding obesity is essential for those with a family history of Type II. Excess weight is the single most common factor in this form of diabetes. And in the majority of cases, the cause of overweight is straightforward: more food is being consumed than the body needs for energy.

People who are under or at normal weight because they have an eating disorder such as anorexia (virtual self-imposed starvation) or bulimia (binging, then purging) also put themselves at risk: they have thrown off their metabolism, upset their hormonal balance, and probably are lacking major nutrients as well.

For those seeking to improve their health and increase their longevity, *what* is eaten is important as well. Selecting nutritious foods over those that are nutrient-poor is one way to safeguard your health. For people susceptible to diabetes, certain foods may also play a part in whether they ever manifest the disease.

The most convincing evidence of this is provided by the Pima Indians of Arizona. For centuries these Native Americans reaped the harvest of the desert—prickly pears, mesquite pods, tepary beans, acorns, corn, and other indigenous foods either cultivated or gathered from the wild. Though theirs was a precarious feast-or-famine existence, these people were extremely healthy, according to accounts written at the beginning of this century. But around 1940, cases of diabetes, usually Type II, began being reported. Today about half of all Pimas over 35 will develop the disease.

Why the sudden appearance of diabetes? Scientists believe that the Pimas' problems emerged when they began to develop a taste for and accessibility to junk food and instant pudding, hamburgers, and white bread. Adapting to a typical high-fat, high-sugar Caucasian diet left them vulnerable to their genetic predisposition to the disease. To prove the point, traditional Pima foods were served to healthy individuals and their bodies' response was measured. The starchy tribal cuisine slowed the digestion of carbohydrates, lowering insulin production and blood-sugar levels.

Daily consumption of mesquite pods may not be the practical solution for everyone who is susceptible to diabetes. But more common foods—mostly complex carbohydrates—do have a steadying effect on blood sugar. Researchers such as Dr. David J. A. Jenkins and colleagues at the University of Toronto have been trying to establish a glycemic index—a measurement of certain foods' effects on blood glucose, by comparing them to the effect of pure glucose.

Originally, complex carbohydrates were considered

"slow" sugars, because it usually takes longer for them to be broken down into fuel glucose; the body absorbs them more slowly and thus blood sugar does not rise as rapidly. Simple sugars like table sugar and fructose were thought to be "fast"—digested quickly, with an equally quick jump in blood glucose. While developing the glycemic index, however, it was discovered that more was involved than just the type of carbohydrate.

In the chart at right, the higher-percentage foods seem to produce the greatest rise in glucose; for lower numbers, the blood-sugar increase is more gradual and lower. As you can see, though, potato—a complex starch—gives a greater boost to blood glucose than ice cream! The conclusion is that the fats in the dessert somehow slow down the sugary effect.

Still, the glycemic index cannot be used to formulate a truly "diabetic" diet. Since the studies were performed on healthy individuals under laboratory conditions, it is not known how these percentages would hold up in meals that include a variety of foods or how they would interact to produce their effect on blood sugar. The food's fiber content and the medications a person may be taking can also influence the results. So far, the glycemic index remains a research tool. However, those who already have diabetes sometimes compile their own index: by measuring blood sugar with a self-testing kit one hour after eating a particular food, they can keep track of which foods have the most adverse effect on their glucose levels.

EATING RIGHT

However, we don't need to know the glycemic effect of every food in order to prevent disease. Anyone who wants good health can follow the "Dietary Guidelines for Americans" issued by the U.S. Department of Health and Human Services and the Department of Agriculture. They're just what

Glycemic Index*

100%

Glucose

80–89%

Cornflakes
Carrots§
Parsnips§
Potatoes (instant mashed)
Maltose
Honey

70–79%

Bread (wholemeal)
Millet
Rice (white)
Weetabix
Broad beans (fresh)§
Potatoes (new)
Rutabaga

60–69%

Bread (white)
Rice (brown)
Muesli
Shredded Wheat
"Ryvita"
Water biscuits
Beetroot§
Bananas
Raisins
Mars bar

50–59%

Buckwheat
Spaghetti (white)
Sweetcorn
All-bran

Digestive biscuits
Oatmeal biscuits
"Rich Tea" biscuits
Peas (frozen)
Yams
Sucrose
Potato chips

40–49%

Spaghetti (wholemeal)
Porridge oats
Potatoes (sweet)
Beans (canned navy)
Peas (dried)
Oranges
Orange juice

30–39%

Butter beans
Haricot beans
Blackeye peas
Chick peas
Apples (Golden Delicious)
Ice cream
Milk (skim)
Milk (whole)
Yoghurt
Tomato soup

20–29%

Kidney beans
Lentils
Fructose

10–19%

Soya beans
Soya beans (canned)
Peanuts

---

*Data from normal individuals (after Jenkins et al., *American Journal of Clinical Nutrition*, 1981).
§25-g carbohydrate proteins tested.

In this chart, pure sugar is listed under the 100 percent heading. Other foods are listed comparatively as to how they raise the blood-sugar level.

the doctor ordered for those of us who may be vulnerable to diabetes.

Eat a Variety of Foods: In addition to the 12 essential vitamins, the body requires certain minerals and trace elements. The only way to ensure that you're getting all that you need is to vary your menu. Include different green leafy vegetables; yellow or orange vegetables; citrus fruits (high in vitamin C); whole grains and breads; lean meats, poultry, and seafood; low-fat dairy products. Taking vitamin supplements is not an alternative to well-balanced eating; the body uses best those nutrients it gets in natural combinations from food.

Maintain Desirable Weight: "Desirable" does not mean the model-thin images projected from the television screen. Rather, it's the weight that has been shown to assure optimum health and longevity, based on your height, sex, and build. To estimate your ideal weight: adult females should allow 100 pounds for the first 5 feet of their height, then add 5 pounds for each inch over 5 feet (or subtract 5 for each inch under); adult males, 106 pounds for the first 5 feet, then 5 pounds for each additional inch.

A small-boned adult should subtract 10 percent from this figure; add 10 percent for a large frame. (A quick test of frame size: lightly encircle one wrist with the thumb and forefinger of the other hand. If, without straining or pinching the skin, the fingertips touch, you have a medium frame; if fingers overlap, a small frame; if they don't touch, your frame is large.) Thus, a 5-foot 4-inch woman of slight build should weigh around 108 pounds; a large-boned 6-foot 1-inch man, 202 pounds.

Avoid Too Much Fat, Saturated Fat, and Cholesterol: Regardless of its source, fat is higher in calories per gram (9) than any other food group (proteins and carbohydrates both have 4). If you're overweight and at risk for diabetes, fats should be your natural enemy, since they offer less nutrition and are less filling at more than twice the calories of other fuel sources.

Some dietary fat is necessary, as it provides energy, carries vitamins A, D, E, and K, and keeps skin healthy. When part of a meal, fat slows digestion, preventing rapid rises in blood glucose. However, a high-fat diet can make insulin less effective. Most of us eat too much fat and of the wrong kind. Those from animal sources—meat fat, butter, cheeses, milk, lard, solid shortening—and from some plants—palm, palm-kernel, and coconut oils—are called saturated fats. They raise cholesterol levels and increase the risk of heart disease. Unsaturated fats, though as high in calories, have no harmful effect on the cardiovascular system. In fact, most will lower blood-cholesterol levels. These fats are divided into monounsaturates (canola, olive, and peanut oils) and polyunsaturates (corn, cottonseed, rapeseed, safflower, soybean, and sunflower oils). Beware, though: vegetable oils that have been "hydrogenated"—as is the case for most stick margarines—become more saturated and less desirable in a diet.

Diabetes has been associated with high cholesterol and triglycerides—both fatlike substances in the blood. Though it's the saturated fat rather than the cholesterol we eat that usually raises our blood-cholesterol levels, health guidelines call for a reduction in ingested cholesterol because the body already manufactures all it needs. Excess cholesterol, whether derived from food or made in the body, can cling to the vessel walls, resulting in arteriosclerosis (hardening of the arteries), restricting blood flow, and making a heart attack or stroke more likely.

Any animal product, but particularly egg yolks and organ meats, contains cholesterol. The amount in one

yolk—275 milligrams—nearly meets the daily recommended limit of 300 milligrams. The chart below lists the
amount of cholesterol and saturated fat in some foods.

Food	Cholesterol	Saturated Fat
Egg yolk	275 mg/oz	1.7 gm/oz
Egg white	0 mg/oz	0 gm/oz
Meat (trimmed of visible fat)		
Beef	25 mg/oz	1.6 gm/oz
Brain	606 mg/oz	*
Chicken, no skin	24 mg/oz	0.5 gm/oz
Kidney	114 mg/oz	*
Lamb	27 mg/oz	1.15 gm/oz
Liver	124 mg/oz	0.83 gm/oz
Pork	25 mg/oz	1.6 gm/oz
Sweetbreads	132 mg/oz	*
Veal	27 mg/oz	0.2 gm/oz
Dairy Products		
Butter	10 mg/tsp	2.4 gm/tsp
Cheddar cheese	30 mg/oz	6.0 gm/oz
Cottage cheese (creamed)	8 mg/¼ cup	6.4 gm/¼ cup
Cream cheese	31 mg/oz	6.2 gm/oz
Ice cream	35 mg/½ cup	5.9 gm/½ cup
Skim milk	6 mg/cup	0.4 gm/cup
Whole milk	34 mg/cup	5.0 gm/cup

*Data not available or unknown.

Avoid Too Much Sugar: While sugar does provide quick
energy, it raises blood glucose rapidly and drops it just as
suddenly. As mentioned previously, diabetes is *not* caused
by eating too much sugar—though this was once thought
to be the case. (Many people still call it "sugar diabetes.")
The condition may stimulate a desire for sweets because,
since cells are not getting enough glucose, the body may
have an unsatisfiable craving for sugar's quick energy. For

those who have diabetes and those who may get it, sugar does not have to be completely eliminated. To lessen its effect on blood-glucose levels, it's best to have it with other foods and space it out over the day.

Still, sugar offers no nutrition, only calories. If you fill up on sugar calories, you'll lose out on the nutrients that other, lower-calorie foods would have provided. For someone predisposed to diabetes, there's the added threat of weight gain when a sweet tooth is too frequently indulged.

Eat Foods with Adequate Starch and Fiber: A leftover from the high-protein-diet fads of the 1970s, the prejudice still persists that "starch" is "fattening." In fact, the opposite is true. Complex carbohydrates—if unsullied by added fats or sugars—should make up the majority of the diet and help in weight control. They improve digestion (and blood sugar), contain nutrient-dense calories, and leave you feeling full—an important factor when trying to slim down.

Those who formulated the early diabetic diets, too, thought carbohydrates had to be limited. Many advocated a high-protein diet, which is now known to interfere with kidney function by sending through too much blood. (Protein is highly restricted in the diets of diabetic patients with kidney damage.) Instead, it has been found that many of these fibrous foods help stabilize blood sugar because they take longer to digest. As the glycemic index shows, however, the body does not respond to all starches the same way. Lentils and pasta seem to elicit a low blood-glucose response, bread and potatoes a higher one. As yet, though, it is difficult to predict which carbohydrates are better than others. Your best bet is to incorporate a variety of complex carbohydrates in your meals.

Fiber gotten from complex carbohydrates takes two forms: soluble and insoluble. The jelly-like *soluble* fibers are pectin (in vegetables and fruits), gums (in oats and legumes, like peas and beans), and mucilages (seeds). They mix with intestinal chemicals to prevent or limit certain substances from being absorbed into the bloodstream. The "woody" *insoluble* fibers include cellulose, hemicellulose, and lignin— found in cereal grains, bran, and fruit and vegetable skins. They absorb water, creating bulk and allowing ingested foods to pass more easily through the digestive system. All plants contain a combination of these fibers, though fruits tend to have more pectin and vegetables are higher in cellulose.

Both fiber types, though not considered nutrients, are necessary for health. Fiber traps glucose, keeping blood sugar from peaking and plummeting too rapidly. In fact, Dr. James Anderson's studies have shown that by increasing fiber, most people with diabetes can greatly reduce their need for insulin injections. High-fiber diets have been linked to a reduction in cholesterol as well as colon cancers. Some fiber sources (oat bran, dried beans, pectins) are able to lower cholesterol, reducing the risk of heart disease—a risk also associated with diabetes. Triglycerides also tend to be lower with a high-fiber regimen.

Most nutrition experts suggest about 25 to 35 grams of fiber (see the chart below for the fiber content of some foods; the American Diabetes Association's Exchange Lists that follow also highlight high-fiber choices). The best sources are whole cereals, such as wheat, brown rice, corn, barley, rye, and millet; legumes, including cannellini or white beans, cowpeas, garbanzos or chick-peas, kidney beans, lentils, limas, navy beans, peanuts, peas; root vegetables, like potatoes, carrots, parsnips, turnips, and sweet potatoes; fresh fruits, particularly berries and apples; and green leafy vegetables. Fiber can also be gotten from nuts and dried fruits, but these should be eaten in moderation as nuts are high in fat and dried fruits high in sugar.

Fiber Content of Selected Foods

Food	Portion Size	Cal	Plant Fiber (g)
Breads, Cereals, and Starchy Vegetables			
Beans, white	½ cup	91	4.2
Beans, kidney	½ cup	94	4.5
Beans, lima	½ cup	126	1.4
Bran (100%), cereal	½ cup	66	10.0
Bread, rye	1 slice	54	2.7
Bread, white	1 slice	74	0.8
Bread, whole-grain wheat	1 slice	63	2.7
Corn, kernels	⅓ cup	41	2.1
Corn, grits	½ cup	59	1.9
Corn bread	1 square	151	2.7
Corn flakes	¾ cup	64	2.1
Crackers, graham	2 squares	53	1.5
Crackers, saltine	6	65	0.5
Oats, whole	½ cup	61	1.6
Pancakes	1	61	0.4
Parsnips	⅔ cup	72	5.9
Peas	½ cup	44	5.2
Potatoes, white	1 small	80	3.8
Rice, brown	½ cup	83	1.3
Rice, white	½ cup	79	0.5
Roll, dinner	1	81	0.8
Rye flour, dark*	2½ Tbsp	60	2.8
Rye wafers	3 squares	64	2.3
Spaghetti	½ cup	82	0.8
Squash, winter	½ cup	43	3.6
Sweet potatoes	¼ cup	72	2.9
Waffle	1 section	139	0.8
Wheat flour, whole grain*	2½ Tbsp	60	1.8
Wheat flour, white	2½ Tbsp	77	0.7
Wheat cereal, flakes	¾ cup	75	3.0
Wheat cereal, shredded	1 large	84	3.0

All values are for cooked or prepared items unless otherwise indicated by an asterisk (*).

Food	Portion Size	Cal	Plant Fiber (g)
Fruits			
Apple	1 small	55	3.9
Apricots	2 medium	39	1.3
Banana	½ small	60	1.3
Blackberries	½ cup	30	3.6
Cherries	10	44	0.9
Grapefruit	½	41	1.3
Grapes	10	34	0.4
Mushmelon	½ cup	26	0.9
Orange	1 small	45	2.1
Peach	1 medium	33	1.0
Pear	1 small	70	2.5
Pineapple	¾ cup	41	1.3
Plums	2 medium	58	2.3
Strawberries	¾ cup	36	2.4
Tangerines	1 medium	34	1.8

All values are for uncooked food.

Food	Cal	Plant Fiber (g)
Vegetables		
Asparagus	15	1.2
Bean sprouts	17	0.9
Beans, string	12	1.7
Beets	22	1.5
Broccoli	15	2.6
Brussels sprouts	24	1.8
Cabbage	11	1.6
Carrots	19	2.2
Cauliflower	12	0.9
Celery	5	1.7
Cucumbers*	7	0.9
Eggplant	17	1.2
Kale greens	16	1.4
Lettuce*	3	0.5
Onions	25	1.6

Food	Cal	Plant Fiber (g)
Radishes*	9	1.2
Rutabaga	26	1.6
Squash, summer	9	2.3
Tomatoes	27	2.0
Turnips	13	1.3
Zucchini	9	2.5

Fiber content is given for the portion size ½ cup. All values are for cooked foods unless indicated otherwise by an asterisk (*).

SOURCE: Anderson, J.W., and Ward, K., *Diabetes Care,* 1978; 1:77–82.

Be aware also that too much processing can strip foods of fiber, as well as vitamins and other nutrients. For instance, canning methods usually involve heat, which can break down fibers and destroy vitamins. Refining—removing the bran from whole wheat to make white flour or from brown rice to make white, skinning or peeling vegetables— also removes much fiber. The idea is to enjoy carbohydrates as close to their natural state as possible.

Avoid Too Much Sodium: Diets high in salt have been linked to high blood pressure, a condition associated with diabetes. The U.S. Department of Agriculture guidelines suggest between 1,100 to 3,300 milligrams a day—that's about one-half to one-and-a-half teaspoonfuls. Check labels on processed foods—most are very high in sodium, which is used as a preservative.

If You Drink Alcoholic Beverages, Do So In Moderation: Alcohol can lower blood sugar—leading to hypoglycemia and perhaps masking mild diabetes. It also raises triglyceride levels—a risk in cardiovascular disease. Current recommendations limit women to one drink per day, men to two. If weight is your problem, alcoholic drinks should be avoided: they're high in calories, while providing little nutrition.

LOSING TO WIN

Certainly, losing weight is the single most effective way to lower your risk for diabetes. Eighty percent of those diagnosed with Type II are obese—over 20 percent of their ideal weight. For most of these people, modifying their eating habits is enough to control the disease. But don't put off slimming down until after the holidays or even until Monday. The evidence suggests that the longer you are overweight, the more likely it is that you will develop diabetes.

Where to begin? Reeducate yourself. There seems to be a genetic predisposition to overweight, but this is very difficult to separate from what is learned about food within the family. Most people's idea of what and how much they should eat began at their parents' dining table. If you grew up having your plate heaped with food or were served meat and potatoes with rarely a green vegetable, you probably re-create these same eating patterns in your own home. You may have no reference for what is considered a "typical" serving portion or what constitutes good nutrition.

To get the daily requirement of nutrients, the average adult should have:

- up to 5 servings of lean protein—meat, chicken, seafood, eggs, cheese. Animal protein is not necessary for health; protein can also be derived by eating grains with legumes or nuts—for instance, rice with tofu; pasta with beans; peanut butter on whole-wheat bread—in the same meal or within the same day;
- 6 servings of bread, grains, pasta or starchy vegetables;
- 2 servings of milk;
- at least 5 servings, any combination, of vegetables (one should be dark green or yellow) and/or fruit (one citrus); and
- 1 or 2 servings of fat.

But what is a serving? You fill your bowl with breakfast cereal every morning. Isn't that one portion?

No, it's probably about three bread servings. To help in portion control, the American Diabetes Association and the American Dietetic Association devised the following Exchange Lists for Meal Planning. All foods are divided into six groups: starch/bread, meat and substitutes, vegetables, fruit, milk, and fat. Specific amounts are given for the foods listed so that, within each group, each item is equal in calories, and in carbohydrate, protein, and fat content. This way, you can "exchange" one type of starch or bread for another freely. For example, you can take your five daily breads a number of ways: a half cup of oatmeal in the morning, 2 slices of rye at lunch, a small baked potato with supper, and 2 breadsticks as a snack; or 3/4 cup of cereal for breakfast, 1 ear of corn with lunch, and 3 cups of spaghetti at night. The choices are yours—and endless.

Starch/Bread List

Each item in this list contains approximately 15 grams of carbohydrate, 3 grams of protein, a trace of fat, and 80 calories. Whole grain products average about 2 grams of fiber per exchange. Some foods are higher in fiber. Those foods that contain 3 or more grams of fiber per exchange are identified with an asterisk (*).

You can choose your starch exchanges from any of the items on this list. If you want to eat a starch food that is not on this list, the general rule is that:

- ½ cup of cereal, grain or pasta is one exchange
- 1 ounce of a bread product is one exchange

Cereals/Grains/Pasta

*Bran cereals, concentrated (such as Bran Buds®, All Bran®)	⅓ cup
*Bran cereals, flaked	½ cup
Bulgur (cooked)	½ cup
Cooked cereals	½ cup
Cornmeal (dry)	2½ Tbsp.
Grape-Nuts®	3 Tbsp.
Grits (cooked)	½ cup
Other ready-to-eat unsweetened cereals	¾ cup
Pasta (cooked)	½ cup
Puffed cereal	1½ cup
Rice, white or brown (cooked)	⅓ cup
Shredded wheat	½ cup
*Wheat germ	3 Tbsp.

Dried Beans/Peas/Lentils

*Beans and peas (cooked) (such as kidney, white, split, blackeye)	⅓ cup
*Lentils (cooked)	⅓ cup
*Baked beans	¼ cup

Starchy Vegetables

*Corn	½ cup
*Corn on cob, 6 in. long	1
*Lima beans	½ cup
*Peas, green (canned or frozen)	½ cup
*Plantain	½ cup
Potato, baked	1 small (3 oz.)
Potato, mashed	½ cup
*Squash, winter (acorn, butternut)	1 cup
Yam, sweet potato, plain	⅓ cup

Bread

Bagel	½ (1 oz.)
Bread sticks, crisp, 4 in. long × ½ in.	2 (⅔ oz.)
Croutons, lowfat	1 cup
English muffin	½
Frankfurter or hamburger bun	½ (1 oz.)
Pita, 6 in. across	½
Plain roll, small	1 (1 oz.)
Raisin, unfrosted	1 slice (1 oz.)

Rye, pumpernickel	1 slice (1 oz.)
Tortilla, 6 in. across	1
White (including French, Italian)	1 slice (1 oz.)
Whole wheat	1 slice (1 oz.)

Crackers/Snacks

Animal crackers	8
Graham crackers, 2½ in. square	3
Matzoh	¾ oz.
Melba toast	5 slices
Oyster crackers	24
Popcorn (popped, no fat added)	3 cups
Pretzels	¾ oz.
*Rye crisp, 2 in. × 3½ in.	4
Saltine-type crackers	6
*Whole-wheat crackers, no fat added (crisp breads, such as Finn®, Kavli®, Wasa®)	2–4 slices (¾ oz.)

Starch Foods Prepared with Fat
(Count as 1 starch/bread exchange, plus 1 fat exchange.)

Biscuit, 2½ in. across	1
Chow mein noodles	½ cup
Corn bread, 2 in. cube	1 (2 oz.)
Cracker, round butter type	6
French fried potatoes, 2 in. to 3½ in. long	10 (1½ oz.)
Muffin, plain, small	1
Pancake, 4 in. across	2
Stuffing, bread (prepared)	¼ cup
Taco shell, 6 in. across	2
Waffle, 4½ in. square	1
Whole-wheat crackers, fat added (such as Triscuit®)	4–6 (1 oz.)

---

*3 grams or more of fiber per exchange

Meat List

Each serving of meat and substitutes on this list contains about 7 grams of protein. The amount of fat and number of calories varies, depending on what kind of meat or substitute you choose. The list is divided into three parts based on the amount of fat and calories: lean meat, medium-fat

meat, and high-fat meat. One ounce (one meat exchange)
of each of these includes:

	Carbohydrate (grams)	Protein (grams)	Fat (grams)	Calories
Lean	0	7	3	55
Medium-Fat	0	7	5	75
High-Fat	0	7	8	100

You are encouraged to use more lean and medium-fat
meat, poultry, and fish in your meal plan. This will help
decrease your fat intake, which may help decrease your risk
for heart disease. The items from the high-fat group are
high in saturated fat, cholesterol, and calories. You should
limit your choices from the high-fat group to three (3) times
per week. Meat and substitutes do not contribute any fiber
to your meal plan.

*Meats and meat substitutes that have 400 milligrams or more of so-
dium per exchange are indicated with this symbol.

**Meats and meat substitutes that have 400 mg or more of sodium if
two or more exchanges are eaten are indicated with this symbol.

Tips
1. Bake, roast, broil, grill or boil these foods rather than
   frying them with added fat.
2. Use a nonstick pan spray or a nonstick pan to brown or
   fry these foods.
3. Trim off visible fat before and after cooking.
4. Do not add flour, bread crumbs, coating mixes, or fat to
   these foods when preparing them.
5. Weigh meat after removing bones and fat, and after cooking. Three ounces of cooked meat is about equal to 4
   ounces of raw meat. Some examples of meat portions are:
   2 ounces meat (2 meat exchanges) =
       1 small chicken leg or thigh
       ½ cup cottage cheese or tuna

3 ounces meat (3 meat exchanges) =
    1 medium pork chop
    1 small hamburger
    ½ of a whole chicken breast
    1 unbreaded fish fillet
    cooked meat, about the size of a deck of cards

6. Restaurants usually serve prime cuts of meat, which are high in fat and calories.

Lean Meat and Substitutes

(One exchange is equal to any one of the following items.)

Beef:	USDA Select or Choice grades of lean beef, such as round, sirloin, and flank steak; tenderloin; and chipped beef*	1 oz.
Pork:	Lean pork, such as fresh ham; canned, cured or boiled ham*; Canadian bacon*, tenderloin.	1 oz.
Veal:	All cuts are lean except for veal cutlets (ground or cubed). Examples of lean veal are chops and roasts.	1 oz.
Poultry:	Chicken, turkey, Cornish hen (without skin)	1 oz.
Fish:	All fresh and frozen fish	1 oz.
	Crab, lobster, scallops, shrimp, clams (fresh or canned in water)	2 oz.
	Oysters	6 medium
	Tuna** (canned in water)	¼ cup
	Herring** (uncreamed or smoked)	1 oz.
	Sardines (canned)	2 medium
Wild Game:	Venison, rabbit, squirrel	1 oz.
	Pheasant, duck, goose (without skin)	1 oz.
Cheese:	Any cottage cheese**	¼ cup
	Grated parmesan	2 Tbsp.
	Diet cheeses* (with less than 55 calories per ounce)	1 oz.

Other:	95% fat-free luncheon meat*	1½ oz.
	Egg whites	3 whites
	Egg substitutes with less than 55 calories per ½ cup	½ cup

*400 mg or more of sodium per exchange
**400 mg or more of sodium if two or more exchanges are eaten

Medium-Fat Meat and Substitutes

(One exchange is equal to any one of the following items.)

Beef:	Most beef products fall into this category. Examples are: all ground beef, roast (rib, chuck, rump), steak (cubed, Porterhouse, T-bone), and meatloaf	1 oz.
Pork:	Most pork products fall into this category. Examples are: chops, loin roast, Boston butt, cutlets.	1 oz.
Lamb:	Most lamb products fall into this category. Examples are: chops, leg, and roast.	1 oz.
Veal:	Cutlet (ground or cubed, unbreaded)	1 oz.
Poultry:	Chicken (with skin), domestic duck or goose (well drained of fat), ground turkey	1 oz.
Fish:	Tuna** (canned in oil and drained)	¼ cup
	Salmon** (canned)	¼ cup
Cheese:	Skim- or part-skim-milk cheeses, such as:	
	Ricotta	¼ cup
	Mozzarella	1 oz.
	Diet cheeses* (with 56–80 calories per ounce)	1 oz.
Other:	86% fat-free luncheon meat**	1 oz.
	Egg (high in cholesterol, limit to 3 per week)	1

Egg substitutes with 56–80 calories per ¼ cup	¼ cup
Tofu (2½ in. × 2¾ in. × 1 in.)	4 oz.
Liver, heart, kidney, sweetbreads (high in cholesterol)	1 oz.

*400 mg or more of sodium per exchange
**400 mg or more of sodium if two or more exchanges are eaten

High-fat Meat and Substitutes

Remember, these items are high in saturated fat, cholesterol, and calories, and should be used only three (3) times per week. (One exchange is equal to any one of the following items.)

Beef:	Most USDA Prime cuts of beef, such as ribs, corned beef**	1 oz.
Pork:	Spareribs, ground pork, pork sausage* (patty or link)	1 oz.
Lamb:	Patties (ground lamb)	1 oz.
Fish:	Any fried fish product	1 oz.
Cheese:	All regular cheeses, such as American*, Blue*, Cheddar**, Monterey Jack**, Swiss	1 oz.
Other:	Luncheon meat*, such as bologna, salami, pimento loaf	1 oz.
	Sausage*, such as Polish, Italian smoked	1 oz.
	Knockwurst*	1 oz.
	Bratwurst**	1 oz.
	Frankfurter* (turkey or chicken)	1 frank (10/lb.)
	Peanut butter (contains unsaturated fat)	1 Tbsp.

Count as one high-fat meat plus one fat exchange:

Frankfurter*	(beef, pork, or combination)	1 frank (10/lb.)

*400 mg or more of sodium per exchange
**400 mg or more of sodium if two or more exchanges are eaten

Vegetable List

Each vegetable serving on this list contains about 5 grams of carbohydrate, 2 grams of protein, and 25 calories. Vegetables contain 2-3 grams of dietary fiber. Vegetables which contain 400 mg or more of sodium per exchange are identified with an asterisk (*).

Vegetables are a good source of vitamins and minerals. Fresh and frozen vegetables have more vitamins and less added salt. Rinsing canned vegetables will remove much of the salt.

Unless otherwise noted, the serving size for vegetables (one vegetable exchange) is:

½ cup of cooked vegetables or vegetable juice
1 cup of raw vegetables

Artichoke (½ medium)
Asparagus
Beans (green, wax, Italian)
Bean sprouts
Beets
Broccoli
Brussels sprouts
Cabbage, cooked
Carrots
Cauliflower
Eggplant
Greens (collard, mustard, turnip)
Kohlrabi
Leeks

Mushrooms, cooked
Okra
Onions
Pea pods
Peppers (green)
Rutabaga
Sauerkraut*
Spinach, cooked
Summer squash (crookneck)
Tomato (one large)
Tomato/vegetable juice*
Turnips
Water chestnuts
Zucchini, cooked

Starchy vegetables such as corn, peas, and potatoes are found on the Starch/Bread List.

For free vegetables, see Free Food List on page 90.

*400 mg or more of sodium per exchange

Fruit List

Each item on this list contains about 15 grams of carbohydrate and 60 calories. Fresh, frozen, and dried fruits have about 2 grams of fiber per exchange. Fruits that have 3 or more grams of fiber per exchange have an asterisk (*). Fruit juices contain very little dietary fiber.

The carbohydrate and calorie content for a fruit exchange is based on the usual serving of the most commonly eaten fruits. Use fresh fruits or fruits frozen or canned without sugar added. Whole fruit is more filling than fruit juice and may be a better choice for those who are trying to lose weight. Unless otherwise noted, the serving size for one fruit exchange is:

½ cup of fresh fruit or fruit juice
¼ cup of dried fruit

Fresh, Frozen, and Unsweetened Canned Fruit

Apple (raw, 2 in. across)	1 apple
Applesauce (unsweetened)	½ cup
Apricots (medium, raw)	4 apricots
Apricots (canned)	½ cup, or 4 halves
Banana (9 in. long)	½ banana
*Blackberries (raw)	¾ cup
*Blueberries (raw)	¾ cup
Cantaloupe (5 in. across)	⅓ melon
(cubes)	1 cup
Cherries (large, raw)	12 cherries
Cherries (canned)	½ cup
Figs (raw, 2 in. across)	2 figs
Fruit cocktail (canned)	½ cup
Grapefruit (medium)	½ grapefruit
Grapefruit (segments)	¾ cup
Grapes (small)	15 grapes
Honeydew melon (medium)	⅛ melon
(cubes)	1 cup
Kiwi (large)	1 kiwi

Mandarin oranges	¾ cup
Mango (small)	½ mango
*Nectarine (2½ in. across)	1 nectarine
Orange (2½ in. across)	1 orange
Papaya	1 cup
Peach (2¾ in. across)	1 peach, or ¾ cup
Peaches (canned)	½ cup or 2 halves
Pear	½ large, or 1 small
Pears (canned)	½ cup, or 2 halves
Persimmon (medium, native)	2 persimmons
Pineapple (raw)	¾ cup
Pineapple (canned)	⅓ cup
Plum (raw, 2 in. across)	2 plums
*Pomegranate	½ pomegranate
*Raspberries (raw)	1 cup
*Strawberries (raw, whole)	1¼ cup
*Tangerine (2½ in. across)	2 tangerines
Watermelon (cubes)	1¼ cup

Dried Fruit

*Apples	4 rings
*Apricots	7 halves
Dates	2½ medium
*Figs	1½
*Prunes	3 medium
Raisins	2 Tbsp.

Fruit Juice

Apple juice/cider	½ cup
Cranberry juice cocktail	⅓ cup
Grapefruit juice	½ cup
Grape juice	⅓ cup
Orange juice	½ cup
Pineapple juice	½ cup
Prune juice	⅓ cup

*3 or more grams of fiber per exchange

Milk List

Each serving of milk or milk products on this list contains about 12 grams of carbohydrate and 8 grams of protein. The amount of fat in milk is measured in percent (%) of butterfat. The calories vary, depending on what kind of milk you choose. The list is divided into three parts based on the amount of fat and calories: skim/very lowfat milk, lowfat milk, and whole milk. One serving (one milk exchange) of each of these includes:

	Carbohydrate (grams)	Protein (grams)	Fat (grams)	Calories
Skim/Very Lowfat	12	8	trace	90
Lowfat	12	8	5	120
Whole	12	8	8	150

Milk is the body's main source of calcium, the mineral needed for growth and repair of bones. Yogurt is also a good source of calcium. Yogurt and many dry or powdered milk products have different amounts of fat. If you have questions about a particular item, read the label to find out the fat and calorie content.

Milk is good to drink, but it can also be added to cereal, and to other foods. Many tasty dishes such as sugar-free pudding are made with milk (see the Combination Foods list). Add life to plain yogurt by adding one of your fruit exchanges to it.

The whole milk group has much more fat per serving than the skim and lowfat groups. Whole milk has more than 3¼% butterfat. Try to limit your choices from the whole milk group as much as possible.

Skim and Very Lowfat Milk

Skim milk	1 cup
½% milk	1 cup
1% milk	1 cup
Lowfat buttermilk	1 cup
Evaporated skim milk	½ cup
Dry nonfat milk	⅓ cup
Plain nonfat yogurt	8 oz.

Lowfat Milk

2% milk	1 cup fluid

Whole Milk

Plain lowfat yogurt (with added nonfat milk solids)	8 oz.
Whole milk	1 cup
Evaporated whole milk	½ cup
Whole plain yogurt	8 oz.

Fat List

Each serving on the fat list contains about 5 grams of fat and 45 calories.

The foods on the fat list contain mostly fat, although some items may also contain a small amount of protein. All fats are high in calories and should be carefully measured. Everyone should modify fat intake by eating unsaturated fats instead of saturated fats. The sodium content of these foods varies widely. Check the label for sodium information.

Unsaturated Fats

Avocado	⅛ medium
Margarine	1 tsp.
**Margarine, diet	1 Tbsp.
Mayonnaise	1 tsp.
**Mayonnaise, reduced-calorie	1 Tbsp.
Nuts and Seeds:	
Almonds, dry roasted	6 whole

Cashews, dry roasted	1 Tbsp.
Pecans	2 whole
Peanuts	20 small or 10 large
Walnuts	2 whole
Other nuts	1 Tbsp.
Seeds, pine nuts sunflower (without shells)	1 Tbsp.
Pumpkin seeds	2 tsp.
Oil (corn, cottonseed, safflower, soybean, sunflower, olive, peanut)	1 tsp.
**Olives	10 small or 5 large
Salad dressing, mayonnaise-type	2 tsp.
Salad dressing, mayonnaise-type, reduced-calorie	1 Tbsp.
**Salad dressing (oil varieties)	1 Tbsp.
*Salad dressing, reduced-calorie	2 Tbsp.

(Two tablespoons of low-calorie salad dressing is a free food.)

Saturated Fats

Butter	1 tsp.
**Bacon	1 slice
Chitterlings	½ oz.
Coconut, shredded	2 Tbsp.
Coffee whitener, liquid	2 Tbsp.
Coffee whitener, powder	4 tsp.
Cream (light, coffee, table)	2 Tbsp.
Cream, sour	2 Tbsp.
Cream (heavy, whipping)	1 Tbsp.
Cream cheese	1 Tbsp.
**Salt pork	¼ ounce

*400 mg or more of sodium per exchange
**400 mg or more of sodium if two or more exchanges are eaten

Free Foods

A free food is any food or drink that contains less than 20 calories per serving. You can eat as much as you want of

those items that have no serving size specified. You may
eat two or three servings per day of those items that have
a specific serving size. Be sure to spread them out through
the day.

Drinks

Bouillon** or broth
  without fat
Bouillon, low-sodium
Carbonated drinks,
  sugar-free
Carbonated water
Club soda
Cocoa powder,
  unsweetened
  (1 Tbsp.)
Coffee/Tea
Drink mixes, sugar-free
Tonic Water, sugar-free

Nonstick pan spray

Fruit

Cranberries,
  unsweetened (½ cup)
Rhubarb, unsweetened
  (½ cup)

Vegetables

(raw, 1 cup)
Cabbage
Celery
Chinese cabbage*
Cucumber
Green onion
Hot peppers
Mushrooms
Radishes
Zucchini*

Salad greens

Endive
Escarole
Lettuce
Romaine
Spinach

Sweet substitutes

Candy, hard,
  sugar-free
Gelatin, sugar-free
Gum, sugar-free
Jam/Jelly, sugar-free
  (less than 20 cal./2
  tsp.)
Pancake syrup,
  sugar-free
  (1–2 Tbsp.)
Sugar substitutes
  (saccharin,
  aspartame)
Whipped topping
  (2 Tbsp.)

Condiments

Catsup (1 Tbsp.)
Horseradish
Mustard
Pickles**, dill,
  unsweetened
Salad dressing,
  low-calorie (2 Tbsp.)
Taco sauce (3 Tbsp.)
Vinegar

Seasonings can be very helpful in making food taste better. Be careful of how much sodium you use. Read the label, and choose those seasonings that do not contain sodium or salt.

Basil (fresh)
Celery seeds
Chili powder
Chives
Cinnamon
Curry
Dill
Flavoring extracts
 (vanilla, almond,
 walnut, peppermint,
 butter, lemon, etc.)
Garlic
Garlic powder
Herbs
Hot pepper sauce
Lemon

Lemon juice
Lemon pepper
Lime
Lime juice
Mint
Onion powder
Oregano
Paprika
Pepper
Pimento
Spices
Soy sauce**
Soy sauce**,
 low-sodium ("lite")
Wine, used in cooking
 (¼ cup)
Worcestershire sauce

 *3 grams or more of fiber per exchange
**400 mg or more of sodium per exchange

Combination Foods

Much of the food we eat is mixed together in various combinations. These combination foods do not fit into only one exchange list. It can be quite hard to tell what is in a certain casserole dish or baked food item. This is a list of average values for some typical combination foods. This list will help you fit these foods into your meal plan. Ask your dietitian for information about any other foods you'd like to eat. The *American Diabetes Association/American Dietetic Association Family Cookbooks* and the *American Diabetes Association Holiday Cookbook* have many recipes and further information about many foods, including combination foods. Check your library or local bookstore.

Food	Amount	Exchanges
Casseroles, homemade	1 cup (8 oz.)	2 starch, 2 medium-fat meat, 1 fat
Cheese pizza**, thin crust	¼ of 15 oz. or ¼ of 10"	2 starch, 1 medium-fat meat, 1 fat
Chili with beans*/**, (commercial)	1 cup (8 oz.)	2 starch, 2 medium-fat meat, 2 fat
Chow mein**	2 cups (16 oz.)	1 starch, 2 vegetable, 2 lean meat
(without noodles or rice)		
Macaroni and cheese**	1 cup (8 oz.)	2 starch, 1 medium-fat meat, 2 fat
Soup:		
Bean*/**	1 cup (8 oz.)	1 starch, 1 vegetable, 1 lean meat
Chunky, all varieties**	10¾ oz. can	1 starch, 1 vegetable, 1 medium-fat meat
Cream** (made with water)	1 cup (8 oz.)	1 starch, 1 fat
Vegetable** or broth-type**	1 cup (8 oz.)	1 starch
Spaghetti and meatballs** (canned)	1 cup (8 oz.)	2 starch, 1 medium-fat meat, 1 fat
Sugar-free pudding (made with skim milk)	½ cup	1 starch
If beans are used as a meat substitute:		
Dried beans*, peas*, lentils*	1 cup (cooked)	2 starch, 1 lean meat

*3 grams or more of fiber per exchange
**400 mg or more of sodium per exchange

Foods for Occasional Use

Moderate amounts of some foods can be used in your meal plan, in spite of their sugar or fat content. The following list includes average exchange values for some of these foods. Because they are concentrated sources of carbohydrate, you will notice that the portion sizes are very small. Check with your dietitian for advice on how often and when you can eat them.

Food	Amount	Exchanges
Angel food cake	1/12 cake	2 starch
Cake, no icing	1/12 cake, or a 3" square	2 starch, 2 fat
Cookies	2 small (1¾" across)	1 starch, 1 fat
Frozen fruit yogurt	1/3 cup	1 starch
Gingersnaps	3	1 starch
Granola	¼ cup	1 starch, 1 fat
Granola bars	1 small	1 starch, 1 fat
Ice cream, any flavor	½ cup	1 starch, 2 fat
Ice milk, any flavor	½ cup	1 starch, 1 fat
Sherbet, any flavor	¼ cup	1 starch
Snack chips*, all varieties	1 oz.	1 starch, 2 fat
Vanilla wafers	6 small	1 starch

*400 mg or more of sodium if two or more exchanges are eaten

The Exchange Lists are the basis of a meal-planning system designed by a committee of the American Diabetes Association and The American Dietetic Association. While designed primarily for people with diabetes and others who must follow special diets, the Exchange Lists are based on principles of good nutrition that apply to everyone. Copyright © 1989 American Diabetes Association, The American Dietetic Association.

The Exchange Lists can help you get a perspective on serving sizes, but you need to know more before you can create your own eating plan to lose weight. You know about calories—the measurements of the heat, or energy, value of foods. And you've probably heard this many times, but we learn by repetition so here it is again: the secret to weight loss is to take in fewer calories than you use up in activity.

How many calories should you be taking in? For adults, multiply your ideal weight (from your calculations earlier in this chapter) by 10. This is the base number of calories needed to maintain desirable body weight. Now figure in your level of activity. Are you sedentary? Do you have a desk job and rarely exercise? Add 10 percent of the base number to the base number. Are you moderately active? Perhaps you take a twice-weekly aerobics class or play a few hours of tennis or another sport on the weekends, in addition to your usual work around the house. Add 20 percent. If you engage in strenuous physical labor daily, you should add 40 percent or more. For instance, if 120 is your ideal weight and your activity level is average: 1,200 + 240 (20 percent) = 1,440. If you're a ditch-digger who should weigh 200, add 800 (40 percent) to 2,000 for a total of 2,800 calories a day.

However, if you are very overweight, you may be eating much more than 1,440 or even 2,800 calories a day without realizing it, and the thought of a drastic cut in food intake may be overwhelming. It may be easier for you to approach calorie reduction with a simpler calculation: it takes 3,500 calories to make a pound. So in most cases, by eliminating 500 calories (for instance, 2 fewer pats of butter, 3 ounces less of steak, switching from whole milk to skim) from what you already eat each day, you should lose an average of 1 pound a week—a gradual but sensible loss.

If you reduce calories too stringently in an attempt to speed weight loss, you could face several problems. When you consume less than 1,200 calories a day, you may be neglecting major nutrients. Also, too little food intake can convince your body that it is starving: metabolism will slow down in the body's effort to conserve energy; you will no longer lose weight, despite the low number of calories you are taking in; and when you resume normal eating, you will quickly regain that weight—and possibly more.

Calories aren't the only consideration when planning a weight-loss regimen. As was discussed earlier in this chapter, some calories are better than others. You could get all your daily calories by eating one pint of premium ice cream and nothing else—and many people do use this "substitution" method as a form of "weight control": "If I don't have dinner, I can eat this candy." But when you're trying to lose weight, your hunger won't be satisfied if you exchange a three-course meal for a 2-ounce bar of chocolate—at least, not for long.

Dietary guidelines recommend that up to 55 to 60 percent of daily calories come from complex carbohydrates, less than 30 percent from fat (less than 10 percent saturated, 6 to 8 percent polyunsaturated, and the remainder monounsaturated), and the remainder from protein. (The typical American diet is fat- and sugar-heavy—about 42 percent fat, 12 percent protein, and 46 percent carbohydrate, of which 24 percent is simple sugar.)

Using these guidelines and the calorie counts for each food group in the American Diabetes Association's Exchange Lists, a 1,300 calorie-a-day diet can be broken down as a total of 6 starches/breads, 4 meats, 2 milk, 3 fats, 3 vegetables (at least) and 2 fruits a day—about 61 percent carbohydrate, 22 percent protein and 17 percent fat. From this, you can mix and match from the Exchange Lists to create a variety of daily menus, for instance:

Breakfast	**Exchanges**
1 whole-wheat English muffin	2 Breads
1 teaspoon butter	1 Fat
1 orange	1 Fruit
Coffee with ½ cup skim milk	½ Milk
Lunch	
1 ounce tuna, mixed with	1 Meat
1½ teaspoons reduced-calorie mayonnaise on	½ Fat
2 slices rye bread	2 Breads
1 cup carrot and celery sticks	1 Vegetable

Afternoon snack

1 cup plain low-fat yogurt, with	1 Milk
¾ cups blueberries	1 Fruit

Dinner

Salad of romaine lettuce, cucumber, radishes with 2 tablespoons low-calorie dressing	Free
3 ounces broiled flank steak	3 Meat
½ cup mushrooms sauteed in	Free
1 teaspoon olive oil	1 Fat
½ cup broccoli	1 Vegetable
1 piece corn on the cob with	1 Bread
1½ teaspoons diet margarine	½ Fat
Coffee with ½ cup milk	½ Milk

Evening snack

3 cups air-popped popcorn sprinkled with chili powder	1 Bread Free

Before beginning any diet, though, you should consult with your doctor. You might also consider talking to a dietitian, who can help you tailor your menus to your particular nutritional needs and show you how you can incorporate favorite foods into your plan. Also, children, pregnant women, and nursing mothers have calorie and nutrition requirements very different from those of other adults, and their eating plans should be supervised by a physician knowledgeable in nutrition and/or a dietitian.

READING LABELS

You can't tell a food product by its cover. If you are trying to eat healthier or lose weight, don't rely on packaging to tell you what is good for you. Bold claims can be misleading. For instance, some products fried in vegetable oil can truthfully be labeled "no cholesterol," because they never contained any—but they still pack too many calories and fat. Beware of other fine print.

Calories vs. Fat Grams: Some "low-fat" products may have less fat then the regular version, yet still get a high percentage of their calories in fat. Remember that each fat gram contains 9 calories. For instance, an ounce of potato chips has 150 calories but 90 of those calories come from fat (10 grams); that's 60 percent fat. The same weight of pretzels has 110 calories and only 2 grams (18 calories) of fat—16 percent.

Serving Sizes: When comparing brands for calorie and fat counts, be sure both products relate to the same serving size. Some manufacturers may call a portion 1 ounce, another ¾ ounce. And even these sizes may not fit into the recommended portions sizes given in the ADA's Exchange Lists.

"Diet" Foods: In many people's minds, "light" means "low-calorie." However, the term has no federally regulated definition; a "lite" product can be slightly lower in fat, or lighter in texture, taste, consistency—even lighter in color. A "light" food may have the same or more fat and calories as the regular version of another brand.

However, the U.S. Department of Agriculture has ruled that "lite" beef must have a fat content of 10 percent or less. And the U.S. Food and Drug Administration does limit "low-calorie" products to no more than 40 calories a serving per 100 grams (3½ ounces); "reduced-calorie" items must have at least one-third fewer calories than the original food.

"Dietetic" has no official meaning. It can simply indicate that the product has been changed in some way to accommodate a special diet. For instance, it may have lower sodium or be "sugar-free." Yet even a "sugar-free" item may still have fructose and/or other high-calorie sweeteners (see below).

Sugar By Any Other Name: You know that sugar abounds in candies, pastries, and desserts. It also shows up in

surprising places—cornflakes and other nonsugary cereals, salad dressings, condiments, crackers—and under
a variety of pseudonyms. It may still taste sweet, be full
of calories, and abruptly raise blood glucose. Even low-
calorie sugar substitutes may contain "buffers"—minuscule
amounts of another sugar to cut the unpleasant aftertaste.
So when scouting ingredient lists, look out for these sugar
clues: brown sugar, caramel, corn sweetener, corn syrup,
dextrin, dextrose, disaccharide, fructose, glucose, HFCS
(high-fructose corn syrup), honey, invert sugar, jam, jelly,
lactose, levulose, maltose, mannitol, maple sugar, maple
syrup, molasses, rawkleen sugar, sorbitol, sorghum, sucrose, turbinado, and xylitol.

The different sugars do affect blood glucose differently.
For instance, fructose—found in fruit, juices, and honey—
is digested slowly and, unless taken in large amounts
or by someone with poorly controlled diabetes, has less
of an impact on glucose. However, all of the sweeteners
are nearly equal in calories and provide no essential
nutrients.

Low- or no-calorie sweeteners pose no particular hazard
to those susceptible to diabetes, though their safety in general is under question. Cyclamates were banned in 1969 by
the U.S. Food and Drug Administration after studies linked
them to bladder cancer in rats. Saccharin, in enormous
quantities, was implicated in animal cancer also, and the
FDA is still keeping an eye on it, but so far it has a clean
bill of health for humans. This man-made chemical is the
main ingredient in most sugar substitutes: Necta Sweet,
Sprinkle Sweet, Sucaryl, Sugar Twin, Sweeta, Sweet Magic,
Sweet 'N Low, Sweet 10, Weight Watchers Sweet'ner. Aspartame, marketed as Equal or NutraSweet, is made from
two natural amino acids, aspartic acid and phenylalanine.
It can cause an adverse reaction in people with phenylketonuria (PKU)—an inability to metabolize the latter amino
acid. Some people report headaches or other minor discom-

forts from aspartame as well as saccharin. Aspartame does not have the bitter aftertaste of saccharin, and it loses its sweetness during prolonged cooking. Otherwise, both sugar substitutes are fine in moderation—defined as no more, per day, than the amount found in twelve 12-ounce cans of any saccharin-sweetened diet soft drink or 17 cans containing aspartame.

Separating the Wheat from the Chaff: When buying whole-wheat foods, look for "whole-wheat" or "whole-grain flour" on the label. Some manufacturers may list "wheat flour"—a sneaky way of saying white flour—and darken the product with molasses or caramel coloring.

MAKING CHANGES

When you decide to lose weight or just eat healthier, don't plan a complete overhaul of your life-style. Gradually introduce new foods and new ways of preparation into your family menus. Otherwise, the temptation to abandon all your efforts will just be too great when they meet resistance by others or don't appeal to your taste.

The greatest struggle in weight loss is in keeping it off. That accounts for the high failure rate for most "diets." Instead, you must decide on a lifelong eating plan. And that requires permanent alterations in eating habits, which can only be achieved by giving yourself time to adjust and accept the changes you'll be making.

- Begin by writing down what you eat for a week (or at least for three days, including a Saturday or Sunday). Record everything—from finishing a child's leftovers, to tasting food while cooking—right after you've had it, not at the end of the day. You need to get the most realistic picture of your eating habits to see what you can do to improve them.

- Little changes can mean a lot. If you think you can't

stomach skim milk, try 2-percent-fat milk. Eventually you might move on to 1 percent, and then skim. You may be surprised how easily you can adapt—after a while, whole milk will taste like cream!

- Don't eliminate; substitute. If you eat ice cream every night, switch to a lower-fat product or ice milk or nonfat frozen yogurt. If you must sauté foods, use olive oil instead of butter—it has the same number of calories, but no harmful saturated fats.

- Make weekly, rather than daily, changes. For instance, to cut down on protein and increase fiber overall, plan at least two vegetarian meals a week, such as pasta with vegetables or meatless chili.

- Chart your progress. For instance, keep a calendar just for recording dietary changes, weight loss, improvements in cholesterol level or blood pressure, etc. Also use it to schedule in rewards for yourself—nonfood pleasures such as seeing a movie, trying on clothing that you couldn't fit into before, asking someone else to take care of a chore for you. This way, you'll be able to flip back through the calendar pages to see how far you've come and how many personal "gifts" you've earned.

- Before eating anything, ask yourself, "Am I hungry?" You may find that your response to food is based on habit ("I always have supper at six o'clock"), emotion ("I always eat when I'm nervous"), or some other outside cue ("Everybody else is ordering dessert; I want some too"). By pinpointing your reasons for eating, you can plan how to deal with them. Ideally, you should wait four to five hours between meals.

- Do one thing at a time. If you want to watch TV, watch TV. If you want to have a snack, have a snack. But don't do both at the same time. Combining food with other activities creates a distraction; you may still have the desire to eat afterward because you didn't pay attention and thus fully enjoy what you ate the first time.

- Don't skip meals. Breakfast and lunch are important to maintain your energy level throughout the day. Besides slowing down your metabolism, missing meals will make you more likely to binge out of hunger.

- Try nibbling instead of gorging. You may find that you feel less hungry if you eat smaller portions more often during the day. Just be sure these "mini-meals" don't total up to more calories than necessary. Research has shown that the "grazing" method lowers cholesterol and trigylceride levels. It also allows nutrients to be absorbed at a slower, steadier rate; the glucose load brought on by eating heavily a few times a day increases the strain on metabolism. Of course, not everyone can maintain self-control if allowed to nibble nonstop, so know yourself; this approach may not be right for you.

- Measure your foods—at least at first. You can estimate that three ounces of meat (the average dinnertime portion) is about the size of a deck of cards or the palm of your hand, but guessing doesn't get you very far in weight loss. Until you become more familiar with serving sizes, you need to see exactly how they measure up on a food scale, or in measuring cups and spoons.

- Get more exercise. If you find you're eating much less than you're used to eating, you can increase food amounts and still lose weight by adding more exercise to your day. This is more than just a trade-off: Activity speeds up metabolism—you'll probably lose even faster. And if diabetes runs in your family, exercise can do even more to tip the scale in your favor. To find out how, turn to the next chapter.

CHAPTER

6

The Exercise Edge

UNLESS you've avoided reading a newspaper or switching on a television in the last 20 years, you can't help but know that exercise is being championed as a cure-all, fountain of youth, and the key to long life. While initially this enthusiasm was taken to extremes, with its promoters recommending an exercise regimen unrealistic for most people, it is clear that regular physical activity provides advantages to health that cannot be maintained through any other life-style change. One of its benefits may be a lower risk of developing diabetes or delaying its onset.

To understand the importance of exercise in preventing this disorder, we should look again to the Pima Indians for an example. Before this century, they, like other Native Americans, took their sustenance from the land—cultivating and harvesting crops, hunting and migrating according to the seasons and the availablity of game. Their lives were habitually full of physical activity. Later, when resettled on government reservations, they had few opportunities to pursue their traditional way of life. A few decades of this markedly more sedentary existence undid centuries of vigorous life—diabetes, previously unknown to these people, became a tribal disease.

This may be the case for many groups that evolved from an agrarian society to an industrialized one. Throughout the economic development of certain countries, the incidence of diabetes has increased as machinery replaces manual labor. When this lack of exercise is compounded by a continuation of usual eating habits, it leads to an increase in obesity—the major risk factor for diabetes.

Studies of two very diverse subjects—Fiji islanders and graduates of Harvard College in Cambridge, Massachusetts—have shown that physical activity can be a boon regardless of ethnic origins: for both groups, diabetes was less common in those who participated in moderate to strenuous exercise than in their less active counterparts.

WHY EXERCISE WORKS

Regular exercise may prevent or delay the onset of diabetes two ways: by affecting blood glucose itself and helping to eliminate other major risk factors.

Lowers Blood Sugar: Because physical activity exerts a substantial influence on how well Type II diabetes can be managed, it is assumed that inactive people are more at risk for developing the disease. Certainly, people subjected to prolonged bedrest are more likely to suffer impaired glucose tolerance. It is well established that exercise improves the body's ability to use insulin, naturally lowering blood sugar. The increased sensitivity to insulin allows more glucose to be taken from the bloodstream, during and immediately after exercise. Some studies have shown that physical training improves insulin sensitivity even in obese patients who do not lose weight. This may happen because exercise increases the number of glucose transporters in fat-cell membranes, and decreases fat-cell size. However, these benefits of improved glucose tolerance are lost when exercise is discontinued.

Burns Calories—Particularly, Fat: Increasing exercise helps in losing weight, a special concern for anyone who has a family history of Type II diabetes. Even minor activity expends calories—using up about 30 percent of your total calorie needs in a day. Once an exercise program is added, this use increases to 45 to 50 percent. A unexpected bonus: Metabolism speeds up for a few hours after exercise; calories are burned at a higher rate even when the body is at rest. Studies have shown that those who decrease food intake and step up exercise lose more weight more quickly. Even better, exercise helps in *keeping* the weight off. (Most people who try to control their weight by diet alone must struggle to maintain the loss.)

The chart at right shows calorie expenditures for common activities. Bear in mind that these are approximate values for a 150-pound individual; the heavier you are, the more calories you will burn.

To get the extra energy they need, working muscles demand the release of stored carbohydrates (glycogen) from the muscles and liver, and fatty acids (triglycerides) from fat and muscle tissue. After you warm up, your body uses mostly fatty acids, then shifts to a mix of these acids, blood glucose, and glycogen. During the early intensity of exercise, the main source is muscle glycogen. As exercise continues, this glycogen is gradually used up and you begin to use glucose made by the liver from fats and, sometimes, proteins, rather than carbohydrates (a process called gluconeogenesis). After about 20 to 30 minutes of activity, most of this energy comes from fat rather than carbohydrates. (The more fit you are, the sooner you will begin burning fat.) Regular exercise, then, will reduce the overall amount of body fat.

Activity	Calories burned each minute	Calories burned in an hour

Light housework
    Polishing furniture
    Light hand-washing
	2–2½	120–150

Golf, using power cart Level walking at 2 miles per hour	2½–4	150–240
Cleaning windows, mopping floors, or vacuuming Walking at 3 miles per hour Golf, pulling cart Cycling at 6 miles per hour Bowling	4–5	240–300

Scrubbing floors
Cycling 8 miles per hour
Walking 3½ miles per hour
Table tennis, badminton,
    and volleyball
Doubles tennis
Golf, carrying clubs
Many calisthenics and ballet
    exercises
	5–6	300–360

Walking 4 miles per hour Ice or roller skating Cycling 10 miles per hour	6–7	360–420
Walking 5 miles per hour Cycling 11 miles per hour Water skiing Singles tennis	7–8	420–480
Jogging 5 miles per hour Cycling 12 miles per hour Downhill skiing Paddleball	8–10	480–600

Activity	Calories burned each minute	Calories burned in an hour
Running 5½ miles per hour Cycling 13 miles per hour Squash or handball (practice session)	10–11	600–660
Running 6 miles per hour or more Competitive handball or squash	11 or more	660 or more

SOURCE: Adapted from Rifkin, H. (ed): *The American Diabetes Association Guide to Good Living.* New York, American Diabetes Association, 1982.

Depresses Appetite: Evidence has shown that sustained exercise keeps the body from signaling hunger. So if you need to cut back on calories, staying active may—literally—take your mind off food, and improve your weight loss.

Increases Muscle Mass: Using muscle makes muscle. During exercise, fat stores are pulled out, while muscle fibers gain in strength and size (though you may not look "bigger," because muscle, although it is heavier, takes up less space than fat). The lower the percentage of body fat to muscle, the higher your level of fitness. (Percentage of body fat can be determined through underwater weighing or by measuring skinfold thickness; both procedures must be performed by a trained technician.) An added benefit: even at rest, muscle tissue naturally burns more calories than fat tissue. Sedentary people who are underweight are just as prone as overweight individuals to be "overfat"—and studies have shown that they too are at a higher risk for diabetes.

Improves Mood: Much has been written about exercise's ability to stimulate the release of endorphins. These natural "tranquilizers" from the brain reduce or eliminate pain and enhance pleasure—they are responsible for the "runner's high" that marathoners talk about. Of course, your self-esteem may improve just from the psychological boost of taking a positive step for your health. This sense of well-being can keep you on track with both your exercise and weight-loss program.

Relieves Stress: Anxiety tenses muscles and exercise un-tenses them. Constricted muscles can inhibit breathing, while activity forces you to take in more oxygen. Sports can also offer a distraction and a way to focus on physical action rather than emotional and psychological frustrations. And don't forget the endorphins—the body's own brand of morphine: their release helps you overcome stress. As you'll learn in the next chapter, too much stress can play a role in the development and control of diabetes.

Strengthens the Cardiovascular System: Like any muscle, the heart gets stronger with use. It then becomes more efficient, sending more blood through the vessels with fewer contractions. Circulation is improved; blood pressure is lowered. Since heart disease and hypertension are linked to diabetes, exercise could offset these complications.

CHOOSING AN ACTIVITY

Not all types of exercise offer the same benefits, nor are all sports right for all people. Planning for activity depends on the results you expect and your current level of fitness.

Exercise can be divided into two types: aerobic and anaerobic. *Aerobic* means "with oxygen"—it increases oxygen needs by engaging the lungs, heart, and large muscle groups. Activity is prolonged and continuous, improving the cardiovascular system's efficiency and endurance. This type of sustained-breathing exercise is also more apt to burn fat, which makes it best for overweight individuals who are predisposed to diabetes. Aerobic choices include brisk walking, cycling, cross-country skiing, dancing, hiking, ice- or roller-skating, jumping rope, rowing, running or jogging, stair-climbing, and swimming.

Anaerobic activities require short spurts of energy, without the need for extra oxygen. This type of exercise tones, strengthens, and conditions muscles, but offers little to the cardiovascular system. Downhill skiing, sprinting, weight-lifting, calisthenics, isometrics, and isokinetics are anaerobic activities. Most team sports also fall into this category because, unless unusually vigorous, the exercise is not sustained enough to keep the heart pumping at levels that maintain conditioning. While not as beneficial in weight loss or overall health as aerobics, anaerobics build strength, which is important for balanced fitness and for improved quality of life, particularly in later years. Being strong means greater endurance in performing even aerobic sports and everyday activities. Weight-bearing exercise also increases bone thickness, helping to prevent osteoporosis, a condition that causes bone loss and brittleness, most often in women after menopause. However, certain anaerobic exercises can increase blood pressure, and should be attempted with caution if you already have hypertension.

Another component in a well-balanced fitness program should be stretching exercises. They can be easily incorporated in the warm-up and cool-down before and after other forms of exercise. They improve flexibility by limbering up ligaments, tendons, and muscles—enabling you to take each body part through its full range of motion, avoiding strains and injury. For flexibility, try yoga as well as simple arm raises, toe touches, side bends, and leg stretches—slowly, without bouncing.

To help you gauge their advantages and disadvantages, here's a closer look at some of these activities:

Walking: This is the easiest, most "portable" aerobic exercise for all levels of fitness, all ages, and all weight groups. It requires no special training or equipment, only a good pair of sneakers or shoes well cushioned for support and comfort. Performed briskly, it gives you the same cardiovascular benefits as running, without the stress on joints and feet. You can sneak it into your day by walking instead of driving, or at least parking a little farther from your destination. Add some stair-climbing and you'll get an even harder workout for your heart.

Running/Jogging: Many people think this is the only aerobic exercise. While it certainly burns calories and pumps the heart, running can stress joints and the spine; if it's not done properly, injuries will keep you sidelined. Good (usually expensive) running shoes are a must to minimize damage. If you're overweight or previously inactive, you're better off walking—it will just take a little longer to get the same results.

Skiing: Downhill skiing requires skill, and provides little aerobic benefit—unless you bypass the ski lift and walk back up the slopes. Try cross-country skiing instead: it's great for the heart, burns more calories than downhill, and takes little more technique than walking. You'll still need skis and poles, though. Snowshoeing is another cold-weather aerobic alternative.

Swimming: This is a wonderful aerobic workout if you're overweight, since the water makes you almost "weightless." It doesn't strain joints, and conditions the large muscle groups in the arms, legs, and chest. You can even take "aqua aerobics" classes—where the water is used as resistance in performing the exercises; for these, you don't even have to know how to swim. Instruction and facilities are usually available, inexpensively, from your local YM-YWCA or community center.

Cycling: Like swimming, biking puts no pressure on weight-bearing joints. Continuous pedaling, with some uphill climbs, pumps the heart and strengthens legs; the upper body, though, gets little exercise. You can take advantage of either stationary or outdoor cycling as long as you pedal without a break and at a high enough tension or gear that forces you to work at it.

Dance: This is the answer for people who don't like to exercise. Whether you go in for aerobic dance (pick a low-impact class to minimize joint strain), ballet, tap, jazz, even belly-dancing, the benefits will be the same and you'll enjoy yourself more by moving to music. For that matter, you can just turn on the radio or stereo and make up your own steps. If you doubt the powers of dance, think of all the old-time hoofers who still practice and look in great shape, well past their prime.

Racquet or Ball Sports: Most are not very aerobic, though if played vigorously they certainly burn calories. Unfortunately, action is often stopped while waiting to serve or otherwise get the ball into play, so you don't get the sustained heart-pumping necessary for cardiovascular conditioning. Often, too, teammates divide the work—and the exercise. (In tennis, singles is better than doubles.) Fewer muscle groups may be used regularly, and if only particular muscles are favored, these sports can lead to overuse injuries. But if this is the only type of exercise that appeals to you, by all means pursue it; you will still get more health benefits than if you remain an armchair quarterback. Begin gradually if you are out of condition, then play more than just on the weekends to increase your workout.

Weight-lifting, Calisthenics, Isokinetics, and Isometrics:
These anaerobic exercises use resistance—a load or weight
applied against a muscle—to build muscle strength and
endurance. In weight-lifting, the resistance comes from
hand-held weights or a weight machine. In calisthenics,
you use your own body weight and gravity as resistance,
such as in performing sit-ups, push-ups and pull-ups. Isokinetics use special devices, including Cybex equipment and
the Nordic Fitness Chair, that adjust to increase resistance
as you apply more force. With isometrics, muscles contract
against a stationary object or another body part, without
moving any joint—for instance, as when you press your
hands together. (If you have hypertension, isometrics may
increase blood pressure; you should consult with your doctor before attempting this or any other strength-training
exercises.) While these activities are not best for the heart
or expending calories, they do improve posture and eliminate lower-back injury by strengthening abdominal and
back muscles. Feeling stronger in general may keep you
active and in good spirits, decreasing your risk of disease.
Any strength training should begin with light weights or
little resistance, gradually increasing repetitions of the exercise before adding more weight. (Increasing weight load
will increase muscle bulk; to tone and trim muscles only,
add more repetitions instead.)

Yoga: It won't help your heart, or burn calories or fat. But
these tranquil movements will stretch and flex you, relieving tension—physical and mental—in the process. (For
more on yoga and stress, see the next chapter.)

STARTING AND STAYING WITH
AN EXERCISE PROGRAM

If you are currently inactive, motivating yourself may be
the most difficult aspect of exercise. It is hoped that knowing it can save your health will be enough to get you up

and moving. The following will help you derive the most benefit from the experience, stave off injury, and increase enjoyment.

See Your Doctor: Before beginning any new exercise regimen, schedule a checkup with your physician. Depending upon your age or physical condition, you may be required to undergo a stress test to determine how your heart, blood pressure, and lungs handle exercise. If you have particular medical problems or take medication, your doctor may also be able to advise you on the best type of exercise, or warn you away from others.

Have Fun: Don't pick an activity only on the basis of how many calories it burns or how famous the instructor is. Your main reason for choosing an exercise is that you'll stick to it—and that means one that you'll enjoy doing no matter what, whether it's ballroom dancing or bowling. If you decide to take a class, sit in on one session before signing up, if you can, to see if you like it. The same goes for videos: rent before buying. Also plan for convenience of time and location; if you have to rush across town right after work to make your class, you'll miss it more often than not.

It's Never Too Late to Get Fit: In a recent study, a group of nursing-home residents in their nineties were supervised in the use of light weights. Every one of these nonagenarians improved her and his muscle tone and flexibility; several no longer needed their walkers. The moral: no one is too old to exercise.

Go Slow: Whatever form of exercise you choose, begin at a comfortable pace, and gradually increase intensity and frequency when—and only when—you feel ready to do so. Don't judge your performance level by anyone but yourself. Never exercise to the point of pain. For cardiovascular health, aerobic exercise should be performed 20 to 60 minutes a day, three to five times a week. Any less than that and you will not reap the heart conditioning benefits possible; any more will add little benefit and may increase your chances of injury. It may take several weeks before you reach even the low end of these goals, but don't rush it. Otherwise, aches, sprains, and exhaustion may discourage you from continuing.

If you feel you can't fit in even a half hour of exercise, spread it out. Some recent studies have suggested that three 10-minute increments a day are as beneficial to your heart as 30 minutes of continuous activity.

Warm Up and Cool Down: Before and after your exercise, always do five to 10 minutes of a slowed-down version of your aerobic activity. (For instance, stroll for a while before speeding up to a brisk walk.) Then do a few minutes of stretching. Your cardiovascular system and muscles need the time to prepare, or unwind, from the work you demand of them. Skimping on this can be a shock to the heart or cause pulled muscles, torn ligaments, etc.

Take Your Pulse: To get the most aerobic benefit from your activity, you should be exercising within 60 to 80 percent of your maximum heart rate. This rate is figured by subtracting your age from 220. Then subtract your resting heart rate (that's the number of heartbeats per minute counted just before rising in the morning). Next, multiply this number by .6 and by .8. Finally, add back your resting heart rate to these two totals to get your target training zone. For instance, a 38-year-old with a resting heart rate of 72 should have a target zone of between 138 and 160 heartbeats per minute (220 − 38 = 182; 182 − 72 = 110; 110 × .6 and .8 = 66 and 88 + 72 = 148 and 160).

To determine if you've reached your target training zone, press a finger to one of your pulse points (the easiest to find are on your wrist, palm up, below the thumb, or on the carotid artery on your neck, to the right or left of the windpipe, just under the jaw). Using a watch with a second hand, count off, starting with "zero," the pulse beats for 10 seconds. Multiply this number by 6 to get the heart rate per minute. Check your pulse before, during and just after exercising. As you become more fit, you'll find that you'll have to increase the intensity of your workout to hit this target range.

Set Goals: They shouldn't be unobtainable, but they ought to be challenging. You don't have to plan to be in the next 10K run, but you might want to make it once around the track without stopping.

Alternate Activities: Plan both a rainy-day and a fair-weather exercise. It will be less boring if you have one more sport to turn to and leave you with one fewer excuse not to exercise.

Do It Right: Proper technique will decrease the chance of injuries and increase the benefits of an activity. If you can, take at least a few classes at first to learn the correct way to perform the exercise or sport.

Dress For It: Shorts and a T-shirt are as good as a designer sweat suit for your daily perambulation in the park. But invest where it counts: good-quality shoes made especially for walking, aerobics, or whatever your sport, designed to cushion and support your feet where needed, will take you farther than bargain sneakers. You'll save on money, and foot problems, in the long run. Also, dress comfortably in loose, lightweight clothing; cotton allows perspiration to evaporate. Wear layers—sweatpants over shorts, sweater over a T-shirt—so you can remove them as you heat up.

Drink Fluids, Before and After Exercise: The body can de-
hydrate quickly, even in cool weather. Water, seltzer, and
vegetable and fruit juices are the best choices; alcoholic and
caffeinated beverages the worst—they're dehydrating.

Bring a Friend: Exercising with a partner—family member,
co-worker, friend, or neighbor—will be more enjoyable and
bring shared commitment. Get your children involved, too,
so they learn the importance of exercise early and lower
their own risk of disease.

Chart Your Progress: Reward yourself for your efforts by
seeing how far you've come. Start from Day 1 to keep a
record of your activity. Maybe you were able to walk only
half a mile your first week and now log in three miles every
other day. Your resting heart rate may be lower, indicating
that your cardiovascular system is becoming more efficient.
Take your hip, waist, and chest measurements: over time,
you will discover that, even if a weight loss has not yet
registered on your scale, you've lost inches—the result of
improved muscle tone and lost fat. These are all positive
signs that your exercise program is working, and will
motivate you to keep going. But the surest sign of your
progress will be the improvements in your health overall,
increasing your chance of preventing or delaying diabetes.

CHAPTER

7

Defensive De-stressing

STRESS is a fact of life. Unless you're a hermit, outside events will have a way of niggling into your conscious or unconscious mind, creating anxiety, nervousness, fear— all the risks of being engaged in the real world. If you have a family, a job, any responsibilities at all, you will feel the strain at certain times. Not all of the stress is negative: starting a new job, planning a wedding, buying a home, or having a baby is a situation that may call upon your coping skills, even though the results are personally satisfying.

Sometimes the source of your stress may not be obvious— an event or emotion long buried may provoke an anxiety attack in a current instance that, on the surface, may not seem threatening. At other times, you may not notice what is producing your reaction—perhaps because you yourself create the tension and avoid paying attention to this fact.

Whether or not you are aware of the stress's source, you register its symptoms. You may feel muscle tightness in your neck, shoulders, or back. You may find yourself clenching your jaw, grinding your teeth, or stammering. You may suffer headaches more often than usual. You may have trouble sleeping—or getting out of bed. You may experience depression, anger, fatigue, confusion, loneliness, irritation, withdrawal, or lack of concentration. A persistent cold or flu, a rash or hives, diarrhea or constipation may be other signals that your body is under strain.

Why do these symptoms appear? They're the result of your body's instinctive physical reaction to alarm of some kind—what is known as the fight-or-flight response. When we are confronted with a stressful occurrence—be it a notice of an I.R.S. audit or winning the lottery—adrenaline is released into the bloodstream. This causes the heart to beat faster. Blood retreats from the skin and extremities—leaving hands and feet cold; it flows instead to the muscles and brain to prepare for physical and mental exertion. Blood pressure increases. Muscles tense. Breathing becomes more shallow. Perspiration increases to keep the body from overheating. More red blood cells are released by the spleen to carry nourishment and oxygen to other cells. Hydrochloric acid is released into the stomach (which, if empty, may sustain damage of the lining and the eventual development of an ulcer). Digestion slows—creating the feeling of "butterflies" in the stomach.

Though these physical changes are meant to protect the body, priming it to confront or flee "danger," stress that goes on too long or occurs too often puts the body under great physiological strain. Eventually, this will take its toll on health. Dr. Hans Selye, a noted stress researcher in Montreal, suggested that effects of stress will be felt at the body's weakest link. If you have inherited a vulnerability to diabetes, stress may break down any resistance to the disease.

In the 1950s, two researchers from the University of Washington School of Medicine in Seattle, Thomas H. Holmes and Richard H. Rahe, developed a chart that gives values to the life changes that create "good" or "bad" stress (see below). Studying a group of naval personnel, they discovered that men who rated high have nearly 90 percent more illnesses than those who had a low score.

In those who already have diabetes, it was found that
"bad" stress—particularly, conflicts with or the loss of a
close relative—had the most harmful effect on blood-sugar
control.

Social Readjustment Rating Scale

Check off each "life event" that you have experienced within
the past year. If an event has happened more than once,
count each occurrence.

Rank	Check if occurred	Life event	Number of occurrences	Mean value
1	☐	Death of a spouse	—	100
2	☐	Divorce	—	73
3	☐	Marital separation	—	65
4	☐	Jail term	—	63
5	☐	Death of a close family member	—	63
6	☐	Personal injury or illness	—	53
7	☐	Marriage	—	50
8	☐	Fired at work	—	47
9	☐	Marital reconciliation	—	45
10	☐	Retirement	—	45
11	☐	Change in health of a family member	—	44
12	☐	Pregnancy (score applies for both spouses)	—	40
13	☐	Sexual difficulties	—	39
14	☐	Gain of a new family member	—	39
15	☐	Business readjustment	—	39
16	☐	Change in financial state	—	38
17	☐	Death of a close friend	—	37
18	☐	Change to a different line of work	—	36

Rank	Check if occurred	Life event	Number of occurrences	Mean value
19	☐	Change in number of arguments with spouse	—	35
20	☐	High mortgage	—	31
21	☐	Foreclosure of mortgage or loan	—	30
22	☐	Change in responsibilities at work	—	29
23	☐	Son or daughter leaving home	—	29
24	☐	Trouble with in-laws	—	29
25	☐	Outstanding personal achievement	—	28
26	☐	Spouse began or stopped work	—	26
27	☐	Began or ended schooling	—	26
28	☐	Change in living conditions	—	25
29	☐	Revision of personal habits	—	24
30	☐	Trouble with boss	—	23
31	☐	Change in work hours or conditions	—	20
32	☐	Change in residence	—	20
33	☐	Change in schools	—	20
34	☐	Change in recreation	—	19
35	☐	Change in church activities	—	19
36	☐	Change in social activities	—	18
37	☐	Mortgage or loan less than $10,000	—	17
38	☐	Change in sleeping habits	—	16
39	☐	Change in number of family get-togethers	—	15
40	☐	Change in eating habits	—	15

Rank	Check if occurred	Life event	Number of occurrences	Mean value
41	☐	Vacation	—	13
42	☐	Christmas	—	12
43	☐	Minor violations of the law	—	11

Total LCU score: __

Holmes, T.H., and Rahe, R.H., "The Social Readjustment Rating Scale," *Journal of Psychosomatic Research* 11:213–218, 1967, Pergamon Press. Reprinted with permission.

SCORING:

150-199   Your resistance to illness is high; you have a mild chance (9 to 33 percent) of incurring some kind of health change in the next year.

200-299   You are at moderate risk (30 to 52 percent) for illness or injury.

Over 300   Your vulnerability makes it very likely (50 to 86 percent) that you will suffer a major physical or emotional illness.

EFFECTS OF STRESS

If diabetes runs in your family, stress can add directly to your risk or increase the effect of other factors. Pregnancy, trauma from surgery or injury, overweight, and malnutrition are all forms of physical stress that have been known to precede the onset of diabetes. Emotional stress can also be linked to some cases; in fact, "stress diabetes" is a specific form of the disease that disappears once the stress is alleviated.

In stressful situations, the body demands more insulin, to let more glucose (energy) enter cells. If beta-cell damage has begun (as it may for those susceptible to Type I), this demand could overwhelm the pancreas's ability to make insulin, and bring on the symptoms of diabetes. The same may be true for people vulnerable to Type II who have already developed some insulin resistance. In one study, a significant portion of the pancreas was removed from a group of laboratory animals; more of those who were then subjected to stress developed diabetes than those who were not.

For patients who already have Type II diabetes, anxiety raises blood sugar. For Type I patients, stress also affects their blood glucose—by either raising or lowering it. Researchers believe that the reason some Type I's react to stress differently can be traced to temperament: in so-called type A (competitive, hard-driving) personalities blood sugar rose; easy-going individuals (the type B personality) had decreases in blood-glucose levels. The type A Type I's tend to produce more epinephrine, a glucose-elevating hormone. Why glucose levels drop in type B's has yet to be discovered.

How long the stress lasts may also be a factor in how it affects glucose levels. Chronic stress—ongoing family or work problems—is more apt to raise blood sugar. Acute stress—such as narrowly avoiding a car accident—tends to lower blood sugar. In any case, someone predisposed to diabetes should try to avoid or limit such fluctuations in glucose levels—by avoiding or limiting stress.

Other side effects of stress can add to your risk of diabetes.

Encourages Overeating: Many people turn to food for comfort, perhaps because of its association with motherly love and family gatherings, or with feeling full and satisfied. Whatever its basis, overeating is a temporary respite from stress that can contribute to permanent health problems. Excessive weight gain means a greater risk of diabetes. The psychological consequences of lowered self-esteem and added guilt can lead to more stress and continued overeating. If you often find solace in food, you need to find a new way of coping.

Affects Hormone Release: As mentioned earlier, the body under stress signals for extra energy. In response, the adrenal glands pour out more adrenaline, also called epinephrine, a hormone that raises blood sugar by stimulating the liver to release glucose. Also from these glands comes additional cortisone, which inhibits insulin, thereby also increasing blood sugar. This can activate Type II symptoms in a person already headed for impaired glucose tolerance. Stress also releases ACTH (adrenocorticotropic hormone), which stimulates the release of corticosteroids—hormones that can trigger Type I diabetes.

Lowers Immunity: Sustained stress drains our reserves of energy. Nutrients such as the B vitamins, vitamin C, and pantothenic acid are continually depleted. Weakened cells cannot fight off invasions by viruses, bacteria, or other disease-producing organisms. And, as was pointed out in Chapter 2, some viruses can trigger an autoimmune process that then leads to Type I diabetes.

WAYS TO TAKE THE PRESSURE OFF

If you're prone to the ups and downs of stress as well as predisposed to diabetes, you need to learn how to disarm stress. The following coping strategies require some commitment and time (leaving you less time to worry!) and perhaps some instruction from a professional. However, once you've made active de-stressing part of your life, you can keep chronic tension from wearing you down, and even resist it before it takes hold.

Exercise: Since the stress response prepares the body for physical action, why not give it some? As was discussed in the previous chapter, exercise can untense muscles, improve blood flow, and encourage deep breathing—all of which counteract the physiological effects of stress. Aerobic activity is particularly beneficial. Fitness will also give you more energy to handle problems as they arise, creating less stress. And again, vigorous exercise will release those calming endorphins.

Eastern disciplines such as yoga and t'ai chi—true mind-body exercises—can have an amazing tranquilizing effect. They usually involve instruction in deep, controlled breathing and focus concentration on simple body movements—and away from an agitated mind. All in all, the perfect prescription for relieving stress.

Meditation: This is another Eastern tradition that aims to control concentration. The effect can be achieved by repeating silently or aloud the same simple sound or phrase (known, in transcendental meditation, as a *mantra*), visualizing a single image while blocking out all other thoughts, or focusing on breathing from the abdomen slowly and rhythmically. These exercises should be performed in a quiet space, away from possible interruption, while seated comfortably, for 20 minutes or more. Some people may view this "mental nap" as nonsense, but it works—restoring energy and unknotting tensions.

Progressive Relaxation: Several studies have shown that relaxation training improves glucose tolerance in those with Type II diabetes, and may be just as valuable to those who want to prevent it. In this process, you tense different sets of muscles separately, holding the tension for about half a minute, then releasing it. For instance, you can start by curling and relaxing your toes, then tightening calf muscles and so on up to your neck and forehead. This teaches you to recognize the feeling of relaxation and enable you to re-create this sensation when needed.

Autogenic training is a similar technique, using spoken commands to encourage your muscles to loosen up and let warmth (blood flow) enter. For instance, you might say, "My right [left] arm [leg] is heavy [warm]" slowly, over and over, repeating for each body part. This self-hypnosis can be practiced lying down or sitting on a straight-backed chair.

Visualization: Close your eyes and imagine that you are walking along the beach, hearing the waves crash against the shore, smelling the salt air, feeling the sand shift beneath your feet. Through visualization, you can fill your mind with the soothing image or the relaxing scene of your choice, trying to reproduce it for all your senses. You can take these therapeutic daydreams farther, picturing a "best-case" scenario that may help you solve a particular problem, and thus reduce or even banish the stress it causes.

Biofeedback: Often coupled with relaxation therapy or visualization, this procedure uses electronic monitoring to measure muscle tension, heart rate, skin temperature, or brain waves. The device emits a beep or tone or provides an image on a computer screen that indicates when a person relaxes or tenses. From these cues, one can learn to control these "involuntary" stress reactions. Handheld biofeedback devices are available, but the procedure should really be performed under the guidance of a trained professional. Check with your local hospital or medical center.

Support Groups: Talking it out is one of the simplest ways to dissipate tension. (Studies have found that people with high blood pressure are more likely to have difficulty communicating their problems and needs.) Even better is sharing your frustrations with others, outside of your family, who are in the same situation; their experiences can also help you come up with solutions of your own. Whatever the source of your stress, you can probably find an appropriate self-help group. If trying to lower your risk of diabetes by losing weight, for instance, consider joining a program such as Overeaters Anonymous, TOPS (Take Off Pounds Sensibly), or Weight Watchers, which offer mutual support as well as ideas for behavior modification. If a family member's alcoholism is creating stress for you, look into Al-Anon. There are even classes in stress management itself. Check your telephone directory or local newspaper for these and other self-help organizations.

Psychotherapy: Sometimes your concerns may be so overwhelming or their source so deeply buried in your unconscious that you will need a counselor to guide you to discover ways of coping. This is nothing to be ashamed of; on the contrary, seeking professional help is a sensible and courageous decision that in itself is a positive step toward reducing stress. There are many different types of therapies and counselors, so thoroughly investigate what each has to offer.

QUICK DEFUSERS

The majority of our stresses are short-term—a looming deadline or a last-minute change of plans. However, they can accumulate to inflict the same damage as tension of a longer duration. You can eliminate or soften their impact by counterattacking immediately.

- **Breathe.** Do you find yourself holding your breath when you are tense? Breathing usually becomes shallower when the mind or body is overtaxed. Yet the simple act of exhaling can release muscles—a natural relaxation response. Take a few minutes for some deep, slow breathing—not with the chest, as most people are wont to do, but with the diaphragm (the large sheet of muscle under the lungs). When you inhale, your abdomen should push out; pull in as you exhale (put your hand on your abdomen to feel if you're on the right track). Breathe in through your nose, counting to four on the inhalation, hold it for four counts and take eight counts to expel the air through your mouth.

- **Sleep.** Take a short nap (about 20 minutes) when you need it during the day to help renew yourself. In general, don't add to mental exhaustion by neglecting your rest.

- **Eat properly.** When you are harried, the temptation is to grab food on the run and forget good nutrition. Make it a priority to sit down to well-balanced meals every day. They'll provide the energy and nutrients you'll need to maintain your health in stressful periods.

- **Delegate.** Overburdening yourself with projects, chores, and responsibilities can quickly lead to burnout, piling up stresses. When overwhelmed, ask family, friends, or colleagues to help out instead of trying to do it all yourself.

- **Just say no.** Very often we take on new duties when we can barely tackle the old. Diplomatically turn down a request or invitation that cannot realistically fit into your schedule.

- **Leave the scene of the stress.** Physically removing yourself from the site of aggravation may be all you need to get away from it. A vacation, a drive across town or a walk around the block may give you a new perspective on your problems.

- **Laugh it off.** When life seems too serious, find something in it to chuckle over. Like deep breathing, laughter untenses muscles and stimulates positive feelings. (In *Anatomy of an Illness,* author Norman Cousins credits reruns of "Candid Camera" with helping to cure a disease that was ravaging his body's connective tissues.) So see a

Marx Brothers movie, share a joke with a friend, or watch your favorite sitcom—those are doctor's orders.

- **Ask for a hug.** Our need for touch is a profound one. Infants who are not held or cuddled regularly are slower to develop, intellectually and physically, than other infants. Human contact—a hug, hand-holding, massage—can dissolve tension, defuse anger, and just make you feel good. Actually, it doesn't even have to be human contact—animals are suitable, and willing, stand-ins. Stroking a cat or dog, even watching a tankful of tropical fish has been shown to lower blood pressure—a testament to the calming influence of pets.

- **Take time for yourself.** We all have more than our share of "shoulds." Family, work, and other responsibilities place demands on us that leave little time for "wants." Even the means to safeguarding your health—lowering your risk of diabetes—adds to your list of "shoulds": you should lose weight, you should eat properly, you should exercise more often. So at least once a day, for no less than 20 minutes, do something you *want* to do. Read a book, soak in a hot bath, listen to music . . . whatever brings you pleasure. In the process, you'll find that you've taken care of at least one "should"—relieving stress.

CHAPTER

8

What the Future Holds

IF you follow the guidelines outlined in the preceding chapters, without a doubt your future will be brighter: you will be doing all that you can to lower your risk of diabetes. Of course, medical researchers will continue to work toward a cure for both Type I and Type II, so that all risk will be eliminated. Certainly, recent advances have already helped those who do develop diabetes live as normally as possible.

Remember that the causes and mechanisms of diabetes were discovered only within the last 70 years. In the past 20, we've learned more about the disorder than in the half century that went before. Through these discoveries, lives have been saved and prolonged, and the quality of these lives improved. Every day seems to bring us closer to a solution that will put fewer and fewer people at risk for developing diabetes. Perhaps in the 21st century, diabetes will be discussed only in medical history books—wiped out as smallpox or polio almost was in the 20th. Research being conducted right now is making that a possibility.

GENETIC MARKERS

As was explained in Chapter 1, researchers began their hunt for a cure for diabetes by seeking out genetic markers—a gene or group of genes that is common to those who have the disease and that will definitively predict who are susceptible. In their quest, scientists have recently switched their attention from the DR to the DQ group in the HLA antigens for Type I. Their work centers not only on which gene predisposes someone to IDDM; they also hope to identify which gene may protect against it.

T cells are also under investigation in relation to Type I. These lymphocytes, a type of white blood cell, help other cells recognize certain antigens and initiate the production of antibodies against them. This autoimmune response may be able to be halted by eliminating or reducing these "helper" T cells. One study has identified a type of T cell that invades islet cells; prediabetic mice injected with a toxin that targeted these T cells were less likely to develop Type I. T cells may also be used to distinguish between much smaller "subsets" of antigens, pinpointing even more exactly which antigens make some people more vulnerable to IDDM.

Though Type II has an even clearer pattern of inheritance than Type I, until very recently no genetic marker for Type II had been identified. Now one study has narrowed the search. Dr. Stefan Fajans, a noted diabetes researcher at the University of Michigan, spent 32 years studying five generations of one family with MODY. More than 40 of the 275 family members had this form of non-insulin-dependent diabetes. From Dr. Fajans's data, medical researchers at the Universities of Chicago, Michigan, and Pennsylvania found that the odds are greater than 178,000 to 1 that MODY is linked to and located near a specific gene on the long arm of Chromosome 20. Whether this information can be applied to the more common type of NIDDM remains to be explored.

What happens once the precise genetic marker has been found? The defective gene will be replaced with a healthy one, or a protective gene will be added to the person's DNA. Sound like science fiction? No longer: researchers at the National Institutes of Health have already begun gene therapy for a child afflicted with a rare inherited immune-deficiency disorder. White blood cells inserted with the missing gene and infused into the patient have begun stimulating the growth of the child's own white blood cells and are producing the crucial enzyme needed to stop destruction of the immune system. Currently, such a treatment does not bring about a permanent cure (it has to be performed repeatedly), but the hope is that it will lead to one.

Certainly, knowing which gene is responsible for diabetes can help identify at-risk individuals. From there, doctors may be able to begin a therapy that can prevent or delay the disease in these people. Some of this research was discussed under "Tests in the Works" in Chapter 4. In other research, studies have suggested that immature beta cells may be more vulnerable to antigens than mature ones. At birth, beta cells produce a minimum of insulin and do not respond to glucose, but they are receptive to glucagon and arginine (an amino acid essential in early life). Experiments were conducted on animals that had been bred to develop Type I diabetes. Beginning six days after birth, their beta cells were stimulated to grow so that the cells would be strong enough to fight off antigens. Only 23 percent of those treated with glucose and glucagon and 20 percent of those treated with glucose and arginine developed diabetes, compared with 65 percent of the animals who were *not* treated. Such forms of therapy to the beta cells might someday be used on people known to have the gene for IDDM.

DRUG THERAPY

As discussed in detail in Chapters 1 and 2, several viruses have been linked to Type I diabetes. Vaccines against those viruses could be developed to prevent their occurrence and thus lower the risk of IDDM for those who are genetically susceptible.

Another approach focuses on blocking the body's autoimmune response—the cause of beta cell destruction. Experiments have already begun with various immunosuppressant drugs, particularly cyclosporine. Unfortunately, though about 25 percent of those treated with cyclosporine have been able to discontinue insulin injections for a time, diabetes resurfaces within a year of treatment with the drug. Even more discouraging are studies that show continued use of cyclosporine can cause severe kidney damage. Other immunosuppressants—such as prednisone (a steroid) and azathioprine—have also shown promise, but researchers have yet to find the combination or dosage of such drugs that will safely and effectively combat an immune-system attack. Timing may also be important: in these studies, immunosuppressant therapy began after beta cell destruction was noted. If treatment were given earlier to individuals known to be at risk, it might have more success. This is the basis of the current research using antibody screening, as described in "Tests in the Works" in Chapter 4.

Animal testing and human clinical trials have begun with a drug that may prevent diabetic complications. Aminoguanidine appears to stop the formation of AGEs (advanced glycosylation end products), complex compounds that are created when glucose binds to proteins. The levels of these compounds are higher in people with diabetes. The accumulation of AGEs in the blood can damage vessels, leading to heart disease, retinopathy, and kidney failure.

TRANSPLANTS

If the pancreas is no longer producing insulin, why not replace it? Pancreas transplants have been performed since 1966, mostly on severe diabetics who have already had kidney transplants. These operations have brought about normal production of insulin and blood-glucose control over many years, and improvement in some diabetic complications like retinopathy.

However, pancreas transplants have their drawbacks. The rejection rate of the "foreign" organ by the body is high. Still, the survival rate for a transplanted pancreas is improving: a recent tracking by the United Network of Organ Sharing found that 71 percent were still functioning properly after a year—up 26 percent from a 1980s study. The most daunting obstacle is the need for constant immunotherapy to prevent organ rejection: the potential side effects of the drugs used can be more dangerous than diabetes itself. And as with any transplant, an acceptable donor organ—one that closely matches the recipient's tissue—is hard to come by.

A more hopeful long-term solution is islet transplantation. Animal studies have shown that it can reverse Type I diabetes. By implanting only the cells that manufacture insulin, the risk to the patient is greatly reduced. The possibility of cell rejection and the need for immunosuppressants still exist at this time, but these problems may soon be overcome. Researchers have found that they can alter the leukocytes in the donor tissue that stimulate the rejection response by cultivating the cells at a low temperature. Deactivating antigens with ultraviolet light and injecting amounts of donor pancreas into the recipient are two other methods that have been effective in "immunizing" against rejection of the transplanted cells.

Work still must be done on isolating enough "pure" human beta cells for transplantation. A new automated procedure has boosted the purity of cell preparations from 20 to 25 percent to 70 to 95 percent. With this setback closer to resolution, trials are being conducted on a select group of diabetic patients today that may make islet transplant a practical reality within the next few years.

SOMATOSTATIN: THE MISSING LINK?

Researchers are also taking a closer look at somatostatin. When injected, this hormone, which is present in the hypothalamus and stomach as well as the pancreas, inhibits the release of growth hormone, insulin, and glucagon— resulting in a decrease of blood glucose. It also slows the development of ketoacidosis in IDDM patients who have not taken their insulin.

The next step for these scientists is to synthesize a substance with properties similar to those of somatostatin that would block the secretion of glucagon and growth hormone (implicated in the development of Type I), but not of insulin, for long periods. Several of these substances have been developed that do improve glucose control in IDDM patients, but they must be injected frequently to have a lasting effect. However, they may eventually be developed for use orally— an improvement in comfort and convenience over injected treatments.

INSULIN DELIVERY

Long-time use of insulin, while essential to those who have Type I diabetes, does cause problems. Injection under the skin is an unnatural way of receiving insulin: when released by the pancreas, the hormone is first cleared by the liver before it can enter other tissues; when injected, it bypasses this process, allowing larger than normal amounts of insulin to circulate in the blood. This condition can stimulate the formation of fatty deposits on the walls of arteries, increasing the risk of heart disease.

Until a way to correct the need for injected insulin is

discovered, scientists will continue to look for safer, more effective, and more convenient methods for delivering this hormone to Type I and some Type II patients. Within the last decade, insulin extracted from animals has been made more pure, lowering the risk of a harmful allergic reaction. And finally, in the late seventies and early eighties human insulin was "biosynthesized": synthesized beta cell genes implanted into the DNA of bacteria can "reprogram" the bacteria to manufacture human proinsulin, which is then harvested, converted (using enzymes) to insulin, and purified—a method that ensures an unlimited supply of high-quality insulin.

To improve the body's ability to use such insulin, researchers have investigated employing liposomes (a type of fat molecule) to carry insulin to the liver. Delivered to this site, insulin inserted in liposomes and then injected are better able to help the body utilize glucose; insulin action is also prolonged. This method is most beneficial for Type II patients who must take insulin and are prone to fasting hyperglycemia.

The search is also on for an oral insulin. Encasing insulin in liposomes seems to prevent the hormone from breaking down in the gastrointestinal system; however, the liposome dose needed to bring down blood-glucose levels is 50 to 100 times the usual injected amount—a costly alternative.

A nasally delivered insulin has been developed by scientists in Denmark. Sprayed into the nose before meals, it is more quickly absorbed than injected insulin. The spray doesn't replace injections, but it can cut down on the number needed daily. Experiments are still needed to determine the spray's long-term safety. If the nasal spray is eventually approved, it could become an effective treatment of Type II diabetes, which requires only a basic level of insulin for hour-to-hour control. For Type I patients, however, the spray would not be adequate for the fine-tuning of insulin levels needed.

As another alternative to injections, the "open loop" insulin pump, acting as an artificial pancreas outside the body, has been in use for several years (generally for those with poorly controlled diabetes). It provides a steady infusion of insulin, but the patient must "close the loop" by pressing buttons to increase the dosage as needed. Unfortunately, the size of the equipment, the need for careful monitoring, and the cost make the pump impractical for most people. However, progress is being made toward developing a "closed loop" pump: a computerized system that supplies a steady flow of insulin and automatically adjusts to changes in blood glucose. The device would be small enough to be implanted within the body, probably in the portal vein, which feeds into the liver—the route insulin normally takes when released from the pancreas.

These are just a few of the areas under study in the prevention and treatment of diabetes and its complications. All evidence suggests that the many mysteries surrounding this disease, in all its forms, will be solved within the next few decades. Some of the resources given in Appendix 2 will help you keep up on the latest breakthroughs that may make diabetes a disease of the past. In the meantime, the prescription outlined here—nutritious eating, weight loss, adequate exercise, and a reduction in stress—will enable you and your family to enjoy a longer, healthier and more active life—and beat the odds against diabetes.

Appendixes

Appendix 1: Glossary

This glossary defines words and processes often used when discussing or describing diabetes. Most of these terms are also explained, as they relate to diabetes, in other chapters.

adrenal glands: the pair of organs, located on top of the kidneys, that make and release hormones including adrenaline **(epinephrine)** and corticosteroids, both of which affect the body's use of glucose.

alpha cells: cells in the **islets of Langerhans** (see below) that make and release glucagon, a hormone that raises the blood's glucose level.

amino acid: any of the compounds that are the basic building blocks of proteins. A chain of 51 of the amino acids makes up insulin.

antibody: group of molecules the body produces to combat a foreign substance or infecting agent (such as an antigen or virus) by weakening, destroying, or neutralizing it.

antigen: a substance or organism, usually containing a protein coating, that stimulates the body's immune system to produce an antibody.

aspartame: a very-low-calorie, synthetic sweetener, made from two natural amino acids and marketed as NutraSweet or Equal. It can cause an adverse reaction in people who have phenylketonuria (PKU), an inability to metabolize the amino acid phenylalanine.

autoimmune reaction: caused by the body producing antibodies that attack its own tissues. It is believed that this is what destroys the beta cells, resulting in Type I diabetes.

beta cells: cells that produce insulin and are found in the islets of Langerhans in the pancreas.

blood-glucose test: a sampling of blood taken to determine current blood-sugar levels.

blood sugar: see **glucose**.

brittle diabetes: also known as unstable or labile diabetes, a condition in which blood-sugar levels fluctuate very rapidly from high to low and back again, preventing an individual from performing daily activities.

carbohydrate: the energy source from food, usually sugars and starches, that the body breaks down into glucose.

cholesterol: a fatty substance found in animal products and also made by the body itself. An excess amount can build up on artery walls, restricting blood flow to the heart.

C-peptide: the connecting compound that is left over when beta cells make insulin from proinsulin. Unlike insulin, C-peptide remains only in the bloodstream; doctors can measure how much insulin the pancreas is actually producing when a patient is taking insulin injections by testing blood for the levels of C-peptide.

cyclamate: a man-made chemical sweetener, banned since 1969 by the U.S. Food and Drug Administration because animal tests indicated it can cause bladder cancer.

delta cell: cell in the islets of Langerhans that makes and releases the hormone somatostatin.

dextrose: also called glucose, a simple sugar. Table sugar becomes dextrose once it's metabolized in the body.

endocrine gland: an organ, such as the pancreas, that releases hormones directly into the bloodstream.

enzyme: a special protein that speeds up a biological reaction, such as digestion.

epinephrine: a hormone, made by the inner compartment of the adrenal glands, that aids the liver in releasing glucose and limits insulin release.

fat: a source of energy from food, which the body either uses immediately or stores as adipose (fatty) tissue; it also provides some vitamins and keeps skin healthy. *Saturated fats* come from animal products (butter, lard, meat fat, shortening) and some plants (palm, palm-kernel, and coconut oils), and are known to raise blood-cholesterol levels. *Unsaturated fats* are derived from plant sources (canola, corn, cottonseed, olive, peanut, rapeseed, safflower, soybean, and sunflower oils), and tend to lower cholesterol.

fructose: a natural sugar found in honey and some fruits. Though as high in calories as table sugar (4 per gram), fructose is absorbed much more slowly and does not raise blood glucose levels significantly, unless taken in large quantities.

gene: part of the DNA (deoxyribonucleic acid—the molecule that carries all information for a cell) responsible for inheriting a particular trait; usually occurs in paired alleles (alternative forms of a gene).

genetic marker: the specific gene that produces a distinct trait, used in research. For diabetes, finding such a gene could determine who is susceptible to the disease. Potentially, genetic engineering could alter certain genes.

genotype: a person's complete genetic makeup—the total information provided in the genes (compare with **phenotype**).

gestational diabetes: a form of diabetes that strikes only during pregnancy and may indicate a risk of diabetes occurring later in life.

glucagon: hormone produced by alpha cells in the islets of Langerhans. It triggers the conversion of glycogen in the liver to glucose so it can be released into the bloodstream. The glucose level is then increased.

glucose: also known as blood sugar or dextrose, the simple sugar found in the blood that is the body's main source of energy.

glycemic index: a concept of measuring foods by how they affect blood-sugar levels. For instance, studies have shown that potato seems to increase glucose levels more quickly than rice or pasta. As yet, however, these measurements have not been standardized and are not widely used in controlling diet for those with diabetes.

glycogen: the form of carbohydrates as stored in the liver and muscles. It is broken down into glucose when needed by the body.

glycosylated hemoglobin: also known as glycohemoglobin or hemoglobin A1C, the result of excess glucose that attaches to oxygen-carrying red blood cells for the life of the cell (about four months). The amount of attached glucose can be measured, showing an individual's average blood-sugar levels for the one to two months prior to the test.

glycosuria: abnormally high sugar levels in the urine.

growth hormone: a substance released by the pituitary gland that stimulates bone growth and affects how proteins and fats are used by the body; the increased production of this hormone during adolescence has been linked to Type I diabetes.

HLA: human lymphocyte antigens—a system of genes that appear on the surface of cells and help fight illness. Within this system, scientists have identified specific antigens that are common to people with insulin-dependent (Type I) diabetes.

hormone: a chemical, released by the endocrine glands into the blood, that triggers the activity of other cells or organs.

hyperglycemia: too-high level of blood glucose, which can be a sign of out-of-control diabetes.

hypoglycemia: a drop in the blood-glucose level, which can be caused by too much insulin, not enough food, or too strenuous exercise.

ICA: see **islet-cell antibodies**.

IDDM: insulin-dependent diabetes mellitus, also called **Type I** (see below); formerly known as juvenile diabetes, juvenile-onset diabetes, or ketosis-prone diabetes.

immunosuppressant: a drug that keeps the body from fighting infection; often given to prevent rejection of an organ or tissue transplant. In the case of diabetes, these drugs may be used after pancreas transplantation. Researchers are currently testing them on patients with early Type I diabetes who have islet-cell antibodies. Immunosuppressants may eventually have a role in blocking the destruction of beta cells and preventing the onset of diabetes. However, little data at present has shown promising results.

impaired glucose tolerance (IGT): formerly known as borderline, chemical, latent, or subclinical diabetes, a condition in which blood-glucose levels are higher than normal, but not high enough to be classified as true diabetes. People with IGT have a higher risk for developing diabetes later in life.

insulin: the hormone that allows glucose to enter cells so they can use the glucose for energy.

islet-cell antibodies: antibodies that attack the body's own beta cells. If these antibodies are present in the bloodstream, there is increased risk of developing Type I diabetes. (Also called ICAs.)

islets of Langerhans: groups of cells—including the alpha, beta, and delta cells—that manufacture and release the hormones used in food metabolism. They are located in the pancreas.

ketoacidosis: also called diabetic coma, a life-threatening condition that occurs when the body must use stored fat for energy because insulin is not available. See **ketones**.

ketones: the acidic by-product of fat burned for energy. If these poisonous chemicals continue to build up in the blood, they can result in ketoacidosis.

kidneys: two bean-shaped organs located in the lower back that filter waste products from the blood; they also retrieve some substances that may be usable—for instance, glucose—before they can be eliminated.

lactose: the natural sugar found in milk and milk products.

mannitol: see **sorbitol.**

metabolism: the process of converting food for use as energy and for building or repairing cells.

MODY: maturity-onset diabetes of the young—an uncommon form of Type II diabetes that strikes children or adolescents, usually those who are overweight.

nephropathy: kidney disease, the result of damage to the organs' small blood vessels, interfering with their ability to filter the blood—a complication of long-term or poorly controlled diabetes.

NIDDM: non-insulin-dependent diabetes mellitus, also called **Type II** (see below); formerly known as adult-onset diabetes, maturity-onset diabetes, ketosis-resistant diabetes, or stable diabetes.

obesity: being 20 percent or more overweight (or rather, over-fat) for one's height, age, sex, and body frame—a condition that increases the risk for Type II diabetes.

oral glucose-tolerance test: an examination performed by a physician to determine a person's blood-glucose level after drinking a high-sugar liquid, usually containing

75 grams of glucose. The test is given over several hours and confirms if the patient has diabetes.

overt diabetes: the distinct symptoms of diabetes, such as frequent urination and increased thirst.

pancreas: a comma-shaped, 6-inch-long gland that releases the hormones insulin, glucagon, and somatostatin—manufactured by the gland's islets of Langerhans—into the bloodstream. Also produced in the pancreas are the enzymes used in food digestion and the hormone *pancreatic polypeptide,* whose function is not completely known.

pituitary gland: a two-lobed organ that releases hormones that control other endocrine glands; its anterior lobe produces growth hormone and ACTH (adrenocorticotropic hormone)—both of which have been linked to the onset of Type I diabetes.

phenotype: an observable characteristic, the result of the influence of environmental factors on genes.

polydipsia: frequent, excessive thirst—a sign of diabetes.

polyphagia: extreme hunger—a sign of diabetes.

polyuria: frequent, excessive urination—a common symptom of diabetes.

pot AGT: potential abnormality of glucose tolerance—a classification, for research purposes, that identifies those at a greater risk of developing diabetes because of family history, the detection of islet-cell antibodies in the bloodstream, or other factors linked to diabetes (as discussed in Chapter 2).

prev AGT: previous abnormality of glucose tolerance—a diabetes-risk classification that includes people who at one time had gestational diabetes or hyperglycemia or impaired glucose tolerance, but who currently have normal glucose levels. These individuals are considered to be at a higher risk for developing diabetes in the future.

proinsulin: the substance produced in the beta cells, which divides equally into C-peptide and insulin.

protein: amino acids linked together, which are the building blocks of cells. Proteins also participate in cell growth and repair. Mainly found in meat, poultry, seafood, eggs, and dairy products, protein is one of the three food classes, along with carbohydrates and fats.

receptors: substances on the surface of a cell that act like keyholes to let other substances enter or attach to the cell. For instance, certain receptors link up with insulin; insulin then stimulates cells to take in glucose from the blood.

retinopathy: a disorder involving the small blood vessels in the retina of the eyes. A common complication of diabetes, it can lead to impaired vision or blindness. Laser surgery can often correct this condition.

saccharin: a synthetic sugar substitute that contains no calories and has no effect on blood-sugar levels.

secondary diabetes: diabetes caused by another disease or condition, drugs, or chemicals that affect the pancreas or insulin production—for example, the surgical removal of the pancreas, or excess production of adrenal hormones (a condition called acromegaly).

somatostatin: a hormone made by the delta cells in the islets of Langerhans that regulates insulin, glucagon, and growth hormone secreted by the pituitary gland.

sorbitol: one of three sugar "alcohols"—including mannitol and xylitol—found in plants and used as a commercial sweetener. It has as many calories as table sugar (4 per gram) but is absorbed more slowly in the bloodstream. Use with caution as a sugar substitute; amounts over 1 ounce per day have been shown to cause diarrhea and may have other long-term effects if continued over time.

sucrose: table sugar, the most common sweetener found in commercial products and the one that causes the most rapid rise in blood-glucose levels.

sugar: the class of sweet-tasting carbohydrates that includes fructose, glucose, lactose, and sucrose.

triglyceride: a blood fat, usually stored for energy; insulin helps remove excess amounts from the blood. A high level of triglycerides is common in Type II diabetes and, coupled with high cholesterol, has been linked to heart disease.

Type I diabetes: (insulin-dependent diabetes mellitus) a condition caused by a virus or autoimmune process that gradually destroys beta cells. Because of this, the pancreas produces little or no insulin, and the body is then unable to use glucose for energy. The least common form of diabetes (accounting for only 10 percent of diabetes cases), it requires regular injections of insulin and usually occurs in those under age 40. Total lack of insulin, if untreated, results in build-up of glucose and ketone bodies in the blood, and can lead to dehydration and death.

Type II diabetes: (non-insulin-dependent diabetes mellitus) a disorder in which the pancreas makes some or enough insulin but the body is resistant to it. The most common form of diabetes, usually occurring after age 40, it is more easily controlled through diet and exercise alone, though in some cases insulin or another medication may be needed.

xylitol: see **sorbitol**.

Appendix 2: For More Information

General Diabetes Resources

American Association of Diabetes Educators
500 North Michigan Avenue, Suite 1400
Chicago, IL 60611
(312) 661-1700

If requested in writing, the center will send information on diabetes education and certified educators in your area.

American Diabetes Association
National Service Center
1660 Duke Street
Alexandria, VA 22313
1-800-ADA-DISC or, in the Washington, D.C.,–Virginia
metropolitan area, (703) 549-1500

The ADA offers information, a catalogue of publications and cassettes concerning diabetes treatment and control. The association also publishes Diabetes Forecast, *a monthly magazine chronicling the latest in diabetes research and treatment; it is available to ADA members or by subscription. Check your telephone directory for the ADA chapter nearest you, or write to the address above.*

Garfield G. Duncan Research Foundation, Inc.
Diabetes Information Center

829 Spruce Street, Suite 302
Philadelphia, PA 19107
(215) 829-3426

This public foundation is dedicated to diabetes research and education.

International Diabetes Education Center
Park Nicollet Medical Foundation
5000 West 39th Street
Minneapolis, MN 55416
(612) 927-3393

The center provides diabetes education and training, as well as research and clinical care. A catalog offers books and videocassettes on nutrition, exercise, and specific diabetes topics.

Joslin Diabetes Foundation
1 Joslin Place
Boston, MA 02215
(617) 732-2400

The Joslin Diabetes Center offers educational seminars and publications, including Joslin Magazine, on various aspects of diabetes. The clinic has affiliates in Jacksonville, Florida; Indianapolis, Indiana; Framingham, Massachusetts; Livingston, New Jersey, and Pittsburgh, Pennsylvania.

Juvenile Diabetes Foundation
432 Park Avenue South
New York, NY 10010
(212) 889-7575

The foundation provides information and education primarily for Type I diabetes, and publishes Countdown, a quarterly magazine available by subscription. Check your telephone directory for chapters in your area.

National Diabetes Information Clearinghouse
Box NDIC
Bethesda, MD 20892
(301) 468-2162

Upon written request, this agency of the U.S. Department of

Health and Human Services will perform a literature search and provide a bibliography on any diabetes topic. The NDIC also offers a listing of materials you can send for and databases for computer searches, and publishes the newsletter Diabetes Dateline.

Basic Reference Book

Krall, Leo P., M.D., ed., *Joslin Diabetes Manual,* 12th edition, Philadelphia: Lea & Febiger, 1989.

Diet

American Dietetic Association
216 West Jackson Boulevard, Suite 700
Chicago, IL 60606
(312) 899-0040

The association offers general information for healthy eating and can help you locate a registered dietitian in your area.

The American Diabetes Association publishes several books and pamphlets that would be useful in planning meals for good nutrition or weight loss. Contact the ADA for a catalog with ordering information for the following:

- *Healthy Food Choices.* Includes a mini poster to help in "beginner's level" meal planning.
- *Eating Healthy Foods.* Suggestions for daily food choices using the ADA Exchange Lists.
- *Exchange Lists for Weight Management.* Help in setting your own goals for weight control.
- *ADA Family Cookbook* (Volumes I, II, and III), *Holiday Cookbook* and *Special Celebrations and Parties Cookbook.* Not for diabetics only, these recipes show the way to healthful eating.

Jane Brody's Nutrition Book (Bantam Books, 1982), *Good Food Book* (Bantam, 1987) and *The Good Food Gourmet* (Norton, 1990), by Jane Brody. These three books by *The New York Times'* "Personal Health" columnist offer a wealth of information on nutrition; the latter two provide recipes as well.

Brownell, Kelly D., *The LEARN Program for Weight Control*, Dallas: Brownell & Hager, 1989–90. A good general program for weight control.

For weight-loss support groups, see listings under *Stress*, below.

Exercise

Bailey, Covert, *The New Fit or Fat*, Boston: Houghton Mifflin, 1991.

Cooper, Kenneth H., M.D., M.P.H., *The Aerobics Program for Total Well-Being*, New York: Bantam Books, 1983.

Institute for Aerobics Research, *The Strength Connection: How to Build Strength and Improve the Quality of Your Life*, by the Institute for Aerobics Research, 12330 Preston Road, Dallas, TX 75230.

Rippe, James M., M.D., *The Complete Book of Fitness Walking*, New York: Prentice-Hall Press, 1990.

Stress

National Self-Help Clearinghouse
25 West 43rd Street, Room 620
New York, NY 10036
(212) 642-2944

Offers listings of support groups and referral services.

Self-Help Center
1600 Dodge Ave., Suite S-122,
Evanston, IL 60201
(312) 328-0470 or (800) 322-MASH

A clearinghouse for the collection and dispersement of information on all types of support groups.

Overeaters Anonymous
P.O. Box 92870
Los Angeles, CA 90009
(213) 542-8363

*Based on the 12-Step Program of Alcoholics Anonymous, meet-
ings involve sharing experiences, strength, and hope to overcome
compulsive overeating. Check local phone directory or contact address above.*

TOPS Clubs (Take Off Pounds Sensibly)
4575 South Fifth Avenue
Milwaukee, WI 53207
(414) 482-4620

*The association helps members lose weight through group ther-
apy, and requires physician-approved individual eating plans and
physician-set weight-loss goals. Local chapters can be located
through telephone directory or by writing to the address above.*

Weight Watchers International
Jericho Atrium
500 North Broadway
Jericho, NY 11753-2196
(516) 939-0400

*The group meetings provide a nutritionally sound weight-loss
program and teach members how to modify current eating and
exercise habits. For location of meetings, check your telephone
directory for local listings, or write to the address above.*

Selye, Hans, *Stress Without Distress*, Philadelphia: Lippincott,
    1974.
Selye, Hans, *The Stress of Life*, New York: McGraw-Hill, 1976.
Shaffer, Martin, Ph.D., *Life after Stress*, New York: Plenum Press,
    1982.

Index